Women's Health Matters

Recently there has been an upsurge of interest in research on women's health. Some of the issues to be addressed are clear, though the methods and problems often are not. *Women's Health Matters*, like its sister volume *Women's Health Counts* (Routledge, 1990), is an invaluable practical guide to doing feminist research on women's health.

For people starting to do research, the completed monograph and the methodology textbook can give only a partial understanding of what it is like to do research, and what the problems and pleasures really are. What, for instance, are the pitfalls of obtaining funding, finding researchable topics, and managing research projects? This collection, with contributions by pioneering researchers and practitioners such as Ann Oakley and Sheila Kitzinger, provides accounts of research work ranging from getting the research idea, through obtaining the funding and doing the research, to the practical problems faced, and eventual publication. The contributors all underline the value of qualitative data and women's own experience in assessing and interpreting health issues.

Intended for social scientists, nurses and medical students, *Women's Health Matters* will be of enormous help both to those beginning to research women's health and to experienced researchers. These lively accounts, with their emphasis on the practical aspects of research, provide an excellent antidote to textbooks and manuals.

Helen Roberts is a medical sociologist working at the Public Health Research Unit at the University of Glasgow. She is best known for her work on women's and children's health, and her most recent publications are *Women's Health Counts* (editor) and *Miscarriage* (with Ann Oakley and Ann McPherson).

Women's Health Matters

Edited by Helen Roberts

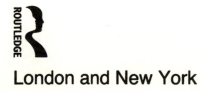

London and New York

First published in 1992
by Routledge
11 New Fetter Lane, London EC4P 4EE

Simultaneously published in the USA and Canada
by Routledge
a division of Routledge, Chapman and Hall Inc.
29 West 35th Street, New York, NY 10001

© 1992 Helen Roberts, the edited collection

Typeset by Selectmove Ltd, London
Printed and bound in Great Britain by Biddles Ltd,
Guildford and King's Lynn

British Library Cataloguing in Publication Data
Women's health matters.
  1. Women. Health
  I. Roberts, Helen 1949–
  305.4

Library of Congress Cataloging in Publication Data
Women's health matters / edited by Helen Roberts.
  p. cm.
  Includes bibliographical references and index.
  1. Women—Health and hygiene. 2. Women—Health and hygiene—
Research. I. Roberts, Helen, 1949–
  RA778.W755 1991
  362. 1'082—dc20   91–12746

ISBN 0–415–06685–9   CIP
     0–415–04891–5 (pbk)

Contents

Contributors

Marina Barnard is a social anthropologist working on an ethnographic study of HIV infection, injecting drug use and AIDS in Glasgow. She has published with Neil McKeganey and Michael Bloor in a number of social science and medical journals on the HIV-related risk behaviours of injecting drug users, prostitutes and adolescents. She is co-authoring a book *Drug Use and the Risk of Aids* with Neil McKeganey which reports in detail on the study. She is currently working on a study on risks of HIV infection among female prostitutes and their clients.

Angela Coulter is Director of Primary Care Studies in the Unit of Clinical Epidemiology, University of Oxford. Her scientific publications have covered a range of topics including women's health, in particular hysterectomy and gynaecological problems; general practitioners' referral patterns; health promotion in primary care; and social class inequalities in health.

Jenny Douglas is Director of Health Promotion for Sandwell Health Authority, and has worked in health promotion for a number of years. Prior to this, she was Research and Development Officer for Training in Health and Race. She has been involved with a number of black community development projects in Birmingham and nationally. She is particularly interested in race and health and the experience of black women in relation to health care. She is Afro-Caribbean and is married with a young family.

Edith Hillan lectures in the Department of Nursing Studies at the University of Glasgow. Having completed a graduate course in nursing, she then undertook further nurse training in paediatrics and midwifery. After a period working in a Palestinian hospital, she returned to the UK and midwifery practice as a labour ward sister. Her research interests and publications include techniques of cervical ripening, a comparison of methods for labour induction, maternal posture during labour, a randomized study of a birthing chair versus the dorsal recumbent position for delivery and the use of information technology in nursing. Her Ph.D. thesis explored the physical and psychosocial outcomes of caesarean section in Glasgow.

Sheila Kitzinger is a childbirth educator and social anthropologist who specializes in cross-cultural aspects of birth and motherhood. She read social anthropology at Oxford, where she carried out research for an M.Litt. thesis in race relations. Her books include *The Experience of Childbirth*, *Women as Mothers* (a comparative anthropological study of mothers in different societies), *The Experience of Breastfeeding* and *Homebirth and Other Alternatives to Hospital*.

Rona McCandlish is a research midwife at the National Perinatal Epidemiology Unit, Oxford. She is responsible for the day-to-day organization of a large multi-centre trial on antenatal preparation for breastfeeding for women with flat and inverted nipples. She has worked as a midwife in the UK and France, and has a degree in English and French. She has a particular interest in women's health and is a member of the Women's Environmental Network.

Ann Oakley is Director of the Social Science Research Unit, Institute of Education, University of London. Her publications include *Women Confined*, *The Captured Womb* and *From Here to Maternity*, and she has recently been involved in a randomized controlled trial of social support in pregnancy.

Jenny Popay is Director of the Public Health Research Centre in Salford, Lancashire. Until recently, she was Senior Research Officer at the Thomas Coram Research Unit in the Institute of Education, University of London. Her publications span a number of fields including work on gender and class inequalities in health and the family, and social policy issues.

Frances Price is a sociologist working with the Child Care and Development Group at the University of Cambridge. She is co-author of *Three, Four or More*. Her recent publications include articles on the medical management of uncertainty, particularly in relation to assisted conception and ultrasonography. She is currently involved in Department of Health research with couples attending assisted conception clinics, and in an ESRC-funded project on kinship and the new reproductive technologies.

Mary Renfrew (formerly Houston) is midwife researcher at the National Perinatal Epidemiology Unit in Oxford where she is responsible for co-ordinating a programme of research studies in midwifery. She has practised and taught in Scotland, England and Canada. She was Chair of the Executive Committee of the Midwives' Information and Resource Service (MIDIRS) for three years. Her publications include *Bestfeeding: Getting Breastfeeding Right for You* with Chloe Fisher and Suzanne Arms and *Maternal and Infant Health Care*.

Helen Roberts is Medical Sociologist at the Public Health Research Unit (formerly the Social Paediatric and Obstetric Research Unit), University of Glasgow, and Honorary Senior Visiting Research Fellow at the Social Statistics Research Unit, City University, London. Her publications include *The Patient Patients*, *Miscarriage* (with Ann Oakley and Ann McPherson) and a number of edited collections including *Women's Health Counts*; *Women, Health and Reproduction*; *Doing Feminist Research* and (with Colin Bell) *Social Researching: Policy Problems and Practice*.

Margaret Thorogood is an epidemiologist with an interest in nutrition. She is a Research Fellow in the Imperial Cancer Research Fund General Practice Research Group in the Department of Public Health and Primary Care at the University of Oxford. Her scientific publications include work on the risk of cardiovascular disease, defects of lipid metabolism, cardiovascular effects of oral contraceptives and the health implications of vegetarianism.

Acknowledgements

Authors of individual chapters make their own acknowledgements, which appear at the end of their chapters. As editor, it is my pleasure to thank the authors, with whom it has been a privilege to work, Talia Rodgers, Kerstin Walker and Bradley Scott at Routledge, and Mary Dortch for meticulous copy-editing.

Like all of those of us who work in this area, I owe a debt of gratitude to the women whose lives and health provide the basis for a book of this kind, and whose health does indeed matter.

On a personal level, I am grateful to the friends and colleagues with whom I have discussed the collection. In particular, my friend Kathy Rosenberg, a Glasgow epidemiologist, was a ready source of ideas, criticisms and jokes until her untimely death in 1990, as this book was being completed. Rodney Barker has provided domestic and intellectual support, Benjy Barker gives me daily reminders of the health effects of motherhood so vividly described in Jennie Popay's chapter, and he, Hannah, Polly, Tom and Rodney Barker are a constant source of pleasure and ideas. I thank them all.

Introduction
Women's health matters

Helen Roberts

There has been an upsurge of interest in research on women's health in recent years, to some extent in response to the women's movement. Much of the research, although by no means all, is carried on within academic institutions of one kind or another. But that this is not merely an 'academic' matter in either its origins or its outcomes can be seen from the wide press and other media interest in women's health issues. Moreover the voluntary sector also plays an important part (for example the Maternity Alliance, the National Carers' Association and the National Childbirth Trust) although most of the researchers will have had some kind of academic training.

But though some of the problems to be addressed may now seem clear, and the way to approach them uncomplicated, research is never as simple as it looks. While traditional textbooks of research methods may seem to give a clear indication of 'how to do it', there are many research questions which remain unanswered by both the textbook, and the polished accounts resulting from completed research. There can be few researchers who have not been struck by the wide gap between the apparently problem-free research trajectory as described in textbooks, however well written, and the realities of carrying out research. This gap is not confined to early work at the beginning of a career. It is not simply a feature of either inexperience or experiment, but is intrinsic to the enterprise of research.

It must be clear by now even to those least sympathetic to feminism that the injunction of the anthropologist Evans Pritchard to fellow researchers to 'behave like a gentleman, keep off the women, take quinine daily and play it by ear' is no longer either sufficient or appropriate advice for those starting research. It is not only the 'stout fellow amongst the natives' view of patriarchal amateurism that has to be jettisoned, nor are the reasons for doing so simply academic. Practical, ethical, social and fiscal problems in researching women's health are matters of public interest as well as of interest to those doing research. And not only does this mean that we should not necessarily expect things to be cut and dried, but that there is real value in pointing out the loose ends and the only partially solved problems.

One such example of loose ends and partially solved problems can be seen in the breast screening programmes, widely promoted as being in the best interests of women, and a funding priority in the National Health Service. Maureen Roberts, the clinical director of the Edinburgh breast screening project for a decade before her death in 1989, asked in a posthumously published article in the *British Medical Journal*, 'Are we going the right way to provide the best possible benefit?' After drawing attention to the limits to the benefits of screening, Roberts further asks the unaskable question of whether screening might actually be detrimental. She points out that one in ten women are asked to return for further, often unnecessary, investigations; that the natural course and treatment of the 10 to 17 per cent of the cancers that are diagnosed as non-invasive are largely unknown, as are what women feel and think about these issues. She suggests, 'More psychological research is required in the screening programme itself, particularly to establish the possible harmful effects on those with cancer' (Roberts 1989: 1153, 1155).

In the presentation and dissemination of research, certainty and numbers are often presented together, and the implication is that they are synonymous. But whilst quantitative methods have their place, they are not sufficient to encompass all the important questions raised in studying women's health, or in studying anything else. The collection of essays in this volume present accounts of research work with women relating to their health, largely using a qualitative approach. Together with the quantitatively oriented sister volume *Women's Health Counts* (Roberts 1990) the book is intended to provide students and researchers with a series of research directions and perspectives which are both intellectually and theoretically sound, but sufficiently exciting to act as a real incentive to those starting to think about doing their own research. The contributors to this volume come from a variety of social science and nursing backgrounds, and the common thread running through the collection is that doing research on women's health is itself a social process and that those who are researched are or should be a part of that process.

This collection is not intended to be read from cover to cover all at once. Different essays will be of use at different times and to different readers. I make no apology here for the relative concentration on a particular stage in a woman's life cycle: a number of the essays concern experiences around childbirth. As Alison Macfarlane points out (Macfarlane 1990: 31), 'Pregnancy is so often treated as an illness that it is sometimes difficult to remember that it is not one. For most women however, it is the first time in their lives that they come into intensive contact with the health services.' This collection is largely about women's *health*, rather than their ill health and the balance of contributions reflects this.

The first essay, by Ann Oakley, looks at the very first stage of a project – the development of an idea, the approach to funders and the difficulties *en route*. The next essay, by Jenny Douglas, is intended to make a contribution to filling the substantial gap in research on women's health which is to be found when examining methodological, theoretical, and practical issues deriving from researching the health of black women. Angela Coulter's and Margaret Thorogood's chapter addresses methodological problems of an issue which many students take up in their dissertations or research projects – women and food. Hypothesis formation is the first stage in any research project, and Sheila Kitzinger's essay uses women's personal accounts to generate hypotheses about the experience of birth.

Moving on to substantive issues described in the context of particular research projects, Mary Renfrew and Rona McCandlish describe some of the problems (and pleasures) involved in setting up a multi-centre randomized controlled trial for and with women. Jennie Popay uses her work on tiredness to demonstrate the case-study approach and reflect on the nature and meaning of women's morbidity, apparently higher than that of men. Ethical issues are addressed by Marina Barnard in her discussion of her work on HIV transmission, while the methodological and practical complexities of a large research project with input from a number of disciplines from obstetrics to sociology are described by Frances Price, in her description of her study of triplets and higher order births. Edith Hillan's work, based on her study of caesarean section in a Scottish hospital, gives helpful pointers to those involved in trying to make clinical audit worthwhile. Finally my own chapter looks at the ways in which we may most effectively use the reflections, ideas and criticisms of our respondents in research.

How might these essays be of use to students, to nurses involved in Project 2000, or to others starting research? To start at the beginning of the research process, Ann Oakley's chapter addresses the problem of how to present research to funders, how to raise money and how to tackle the question of scientific respectability. It focuses on the problems that arise when one is trying to operate within or between two different models of research, a problem which is probably common to a great deal of work on women's health. This raises the issue of the textbook model versus research-in-the-real-world, with attention given to how working in a feminist context gives certain aspects of the research process more prominence than others. It may give some cold comfort to researchers struggling with funding problems to realize that a research and publication record such as Oakley's is no guarantee of an easy ride from funding bodies.

Research work specifically on the health of black women, particularly from a feminist perspective, remains thin on the ground in Britain. Jenny Douglas's chapter reviews such work as there is, and discusses some of its strengths and weaknesses. She looks at the problems which arise when white women carry out research into black women and their health, and speculates on what an ideal research agenda for black women might look like.

The sorts of difficulties which may be specifically associated with such research were experienced by Berry Mayall. She describes interviews carried out by a member of her research team with mothers of West Indian origin about their children's health:

> Women told her that it was obvious she as a black woman must be working as a junior in a white dominated research project. Why otherwise would she be asking questions which lay at a tangent to [their] concerns? Specifically, these women said that what concerned them was racism, housing, finding decent employment and daycare; they were not worried about their children's health and did not see it as an important topic of discussion. Indeed the child, in her unbounding health and vitality, was the principal bright and unproblematic spot in an otherwise troubled life.
>
> (Mayall 1990: 8)

It has already been pointed out that the focus of this collection is women's health, and not their ill health. Ill health and health events such as childbirth give only one part of the picture. In terms of public health however, there needs to be a focus on the wider issues of transport, environment and food. The chapter by Angela Coulter and Margaret Thorogood focuses on the last of these, beginning by looking at why food is an important issue for women's health. It includes material on food and health, women's role in food purchase and preparation, variations in dietary intake and diet and disease, in particular cancer and cardiovascular disease. The methodological difficulties in studying diet are described, and the authors suggest what research in this area can tell us, and why men and women report different diets. Finally, the authors ask what the implications are for research of this kind on health promotion and social policy – a question which many health researchers have to face in looking at the translation of their findings into practice or policy.

Sheila Kitzinger, whose work has been influential in the childbirth experience of women not just in the United Kingdom but all over the world, works and writes from outside the academy, while drawing on her skills as an anthropologist. She begins her chapter with a discussion of research objectivity and what 'counts' as research. She draws attention to the playing down (particularly in the academic enterprise) of emotion as something which contaminates research and the consequent divorce of much research from the lived experiences of those being researched. While professionals are no longer as inclined as they were, particularly in the area of childbirth, to say 'What we don't know isn't knowledge', there remains a deep-seated suspicion of women's own accounts, which are often dismissed as mere anecdote. Kitzinger suggests that female experience, particularly in relation to childbirth, is often ignored or trivialized because it does not match with 'observable facts' or mesh with male ('expert') perceptions of the same event or process. The recording of length of labour and the number of interventions is, she suggests, one way of measuring the quality of the childbirth experience. It yields manageable numerical data. Psychological data are often drawn from a model of childbirth that is essentially based on a medical model. Women are warned not to listen to 'wicked women with their malicious lying tongues'. Kitzinger draws on both the medical and social science literature, and accounts sent to her, to look again at the nature of medicalized childbirth, arguing that there is a well of hidden and painful experience and that aspects of the western way of birth can prove to be another form of institutionalized violence against women. While recognizing that childbirth in the past could be an ugly experience, Kitzinger suggests that accounts of problematic childbirth could profitably be used for hypothesis formation. Meanwhile she suggests that a system of lay referral to birth crisis counsellors can help give meaning and validity to the experiences which women, under pressure to give a positive account of childbirth, may be unable to discuss elsewhere.

In their chapter describing the first midwives' multi-centre randomized controlled trial (and the first, so far as the authors are aware, where service users are actively involved), Mary Renfrew and Rona McCandlish choose to address a question posed by both women and midwives. As midwives have been moving towards working with women more and more (as is appropriate for a profession whose title means literally 'with women'), it is appropriate that the next stage should involve women in running a trial in an area they have identified. That such a trial is complex and not without difficulties is clear, but the authors make a convincing case for the active involvement of women in the research process.

Gender inequalities in the experience of health and illness have been the focus of considerable attention and the overall pattern is now well established. In general, men experience higher mortality than women in every age group, whilst the pattern for morbidity is reversed. This general picture is, however, complicated when one looks at different types of morbidity and mortality and different age groups. This has led to a focus on artefactual explanations for differences in morbidity, in other words, the suggestion that women's experience of minor illness is in some sense not real. It has been argued, for instance, that women are more inclined to report ill health than men, and more sensitive to illness and pain, but that these are not measures of 'real' illness.

Jennie Popay's chapter, based on a number of household case-studies, suggests that these artefactual explanations fail to take into account the meanings men and women attach to the experience of ill health, and neglect the subjective reality of their daily lives. Using the commonly reported symptom of tiredness as an example, she illustrates how listening to subjective accounts can enrich our understanding of the processes which generate gendered differences in the experiences of health and illness. The work on which this chapter is based comes from both secondary analysis of large-scale survey work and a small-scale case-study approach focusing on eighteen London households. The chapter is built largely around the case-studies, though drawing on the findings of the survey analysis. While large data sets such as the General Household

Survey (GHS) can provide an understanding of the range and extent of a number of health issues (see Arber 1990), case-study research such as that reported here can explore the ways in which people attach meanings to good or poor health, and the social structures or processes which shape such meanings. To what extent do high or low standards of living enable women (and men) to reduce some of the less desirable effects on health (such as chronic tiredness) of parenting young children? Popay, in using her case-studies to look at some of the cross-cutting tensions of gender and social class, is able to make sense of the commonality of severe and chronic tiredness across social classes.

Tiredness, fatigue or exhaustion are commonly reported symptoms in studies of women's health (McIlwaine *et al.* 1989). While it may be acceptable, and even expected, that mothers may admit to tiredness, to allow this to get in the way of being a good mother, to allow oneself in Graham's (1982) terms not to cope, is far from being conventionally acceptable. This ability to cope, even under conditions of chronic exhaustion, is explored further in Frances Price's chapter, which is based on work done on the Parents' Study, one part of the National Study of Triplets and Higher Order Births. To conceive, deliver, nurture and care for triplets, quadruplets, quintuplets or more (higher order multiple-birth children) are difficult experiences for any woman. These children are likely to be born pre-term, of low birth-weight, and to require neonatal care. The task of looking after them is very demanding. The first part of this chapter describes the parents' study, early methodological and practical problems, and strategies adopted to overcome these. The chapter then describes the problems faced by those who care for 'same age' infants. Finally, the author looks at the impact on maternal health of caring for three, four or more. The arrival of these babies is an exacting test, not only of relationships, commitments and priorities, but also of the effectiveness of health and social services in providing care.

Marina Barnard's chapter addresses practical and ethical issues within the context of a particular research project. She describes one aspect of a Glasgow-based piece of research on young people's risk of HIV infection on which she was employed as a medical anthropologist, a study of 200 female sex industry street workers in Glasgow. Researching the social dynamics of AIDS and its putative agent HIV raises a variety of methodological and ethical issues for researchers. Many of the behaviours considered a high risk for HIV are socially stigmatized and illegal. In consequence, those involved are difficult to contact and reluctant to talk, and researchers have learned to adopt flexible, often quite eclectic, methods of data collection. A strictly scientific approach to this work might attempt to minimize the interference caused by the researcher. However, in a situation where subjects are at high risk of becoming infected with a life-threatening disease, how ethical is it for the researcher to define his or her role in strictly scientific terms and simply observe or record? In the study described here, the researchers opted to combine a service provider and a research role through offering women condoms or sterile injecting equipment. This chapter examines the combination of methodological and ethical issues raised by this particular approach to data collection. Barnard discusses some of the moral, ethical and practical issues which may arise as part of a research project, describes some of the dilemmas faced, reflects on the mix of pragmatism and flexibility underpinning the research design, and touches on the thorny issue of informed consent in social research.

As Sheila Kitzinger's chapter described above indicates, women's own health experiences and accounts are often ignored, trivialized or explained away. A new twist to this situation is that the current vogue for investigating 'consumer satisfaction' has led to a tendency in some quarters – not precisely to ignore women's feelings – but to 'medicalize' or 'pathologize' them. For women's experiences to be expressed in terms which are both meaningful within some form of market, and amenable to management control, they must be reduced and neatly packaged. Women may be asked to rate on a scale of 1 to 5 the pleasantness or otherwise of episiotomy, acceleration of labour or caesarean section. Women who have recently undergone the experience of miscarriage or stillbirth may be asked to complete inventories on anxiety, depression or their general health. If this is part of the validation of the lived experiences of women describing their health and ill health, there is clearly a place for it. If it becomes merely a curriculum-vitae lengthening experience for doctors in training who are persuaded that 'consumers' are the flavour of the month, then the research itself is in danger of becoming yet another form of institutionalized abuse of women, and misuse of their time.

Edith Hillan's chapter describes an approach to audit and to seeking women's views of a particular procedure and suggests how this might feed into practice on a local basis. Practising nurses and midwives are in a privileged position to listen to patients, although current spending cuts in the health services may very much limit this time. On the other hand, it is important that the politically-led desire of health authorities and health boards to take the 'consumer's' view into account should be seized by researchers and practitioners committed to doing their best to present a real reflection of those views, in all their heterogeneity and complexity, to ensure that the 'consumers' are indeed listened to effectively.

The final chapter, my own, describes something of the ambiguous role of respondents and participants in health research. Without the women who actively or passively take part in a project, there can be no research at all. But they are are none the less frequently firmly pushed off stage in clinical research, and if they have the occasional walk-on part in social science research, are still treated as inconvenient intrusions from the wings. The relationship between what we want to know, and what respondents want to tell us, is frequently an uneasy one. From the randomized clinical trial to the 'softest' of social research on the health of women the respondent, participant, or 'subject' of research is the vital raw material of the research. In the published or otherwise marketed research 'product' however, this vital raw material is normally kept firmly backstage. Reports of clinical trials or case reports in the medical literature frequently acknowledge the part played by doctors who have referred patients. The actual patients, on the other hand, remain unacknowledged for their equally important part in the research. In more qualitative research, the initial bleakness of the statistics may be lightened or their message illustrated by selected witty, unusual or otherwise colourful responses. But it is the privilege accorded to the singing dog or the whistling hen, an exception which, by its quality, both points to the normality of exclusion and, though this is not the intention, calls that exclusion into question for the sceptical reader.

This chapter reviews some of the clinical and sociological literature on the direct and indirect part played by respondents in research, discusses some of the costs and benefits to those respondents, and looks at ethical issues of participation in research. Finally it draws on a piece of research where the respondents were systematically invited to make their own active and open-ended contribution. A final page was added to the questionnaire of a Scottish study, 'Women's experiences during pregnancy'. This provides a glimpse at some of the possibilities for enriching research which can be provided by women themselves, who can never simply be objects of research, since it is, in the last resort, their interests and their health which justifies the whole research enterprise.

The active contribution of the objects of research can no longer be avoided, whether the matter is approached from the renewed interest in citizenship, or the rather more solidly established insistence that services and goods be provided within a market. Whether as citizens or as consumers, women are the custodians of their own experience of health, and whatever the quality of insight which experts can bring to bear, the human subject is always, in the end, central.

References

Arber, S. (1990) 'Revealing women's health: Re-analysing the General Household Survey', in Helen Roberts (ed.) *Women's Health Counts*, London: Routledge.

Graham, H. (1982) 'Coping, or how mothers are seen and not heard', in S. Friedmarsh and E. Sarah (eds) *On the Problems of Men*, London: The Women's Press.

Macfarlane, A. (1990) 'Official statistics and women's health and illness', in Helen Roberts (ed.) *Women's Health Counts*, London: Routledge.

MacIlwaine, G., Rosenberg K., Rooney, I. (1989) 'The health of mid-life inner-city women', *Journal of Psychosomatic Obstetrics and Gynaecology* 10, suppl. 1: 102.

Mayall, B. (1990) 'Researching child care in a multi-ethnic society', unpublished paper, London: Thomas Coram Research Unit.

Roberts, H. (1990) (ed.) *Women's Health Counts*, London: Routledge.

Roberts, M. M. (1989) 'Breast screening: Time for a re-think?' *British Medical Journal* 289: 1153–5.

Chapter 1

Getting at the oyster
One of many lessons from the Social Support and Pregnancy Outcome Study

Ann Oakley

Textbooks of sociological methods commonly assume that research is a systematic, linear process. In this textbook model, research projects begin with a list of hypotheses to be tested and end with neatly data-based conclusions. Epistemological critiques of sociology over the past three decades have posed a certain challenge to the simplicity of the textbook model. But awareness of the need for 'a sociology of the research process' (Platt 1976) imposes on researchers the further requirement of building up a picture of how research is actually done. This 'housework' of the research process includes the genesis of research ideas in the life experiences of researchers, the pursuit of research funding, theoretical, methodological, practical and ethical problems encountered in carrying out the research, and a discussion of choices, techniques, ethics and consequences of research dissemination.

Like housework, social research in many countries is embedded in a culture of impermanence. Contract research as a form of labour thus tends to be sharply sensitive to the practical exigencies of life (see Bernstein 1984). This structural context within which research is done forms an important backdrop to the issues discussed in this chapter. Its purpose is to consider one of the 'housework of research' issues – that of research funding – in relation to a research project concerning the provision of social support for childbearing women. The point of the story is not to complain about unfair treatment from a funding body, but instead to document the process by which a research project moves along the path from idea to 'reality', and to expose the difficulties encountered by research which does not easily fit into conventional models of what research 'is'. The study has been, and is being, written up and published elsewhere (see Oakley 1989a; Oakley 1989b; Oakley forthcoming; Oakley, Rajan and Grant 1990; Oakley, Rajan and Robertson 1990); the story of funding difficulties told here ultimately had a happy ending, albeit one which entailed a series of moral and other lessons of its own.

Although the research project concerns reproductive health, the relevance to women as subjects of study of the wider epistemological and ideological issues raised in this chapter may appear more tenuous. As Dorothy Smith (1987) has argued, there is no 'knowledge' of any kind that is not mediated by the experience of everyday life. Not only are such experiences themselves gender-differentiated, but the *relationships* of men and women to these experiences are also differently shaped by cultural factors (Miller 1976; Chodorow 1978). In the context of social research, it could be argued that women's role as houseworkers, both in general and within the discipline of sociology, results in the insight of considerable disjunctures between the actual experience of research and the model of how research is supposed to be experienced. A sensitivity to the practical and other nuances of everyday life is likely to heighten one's awareness of the 'ivory tower' nature of ideal-type paradigms. The different socializations and positions of male and female in the doing of research interact with one another to produce a view, not only of the gendered nature of society, but of social science. I return to this point later.

Origins

The Social Support and Pregnancy Outcome (SSPO) Study had its origins in six sets of observations, with somewhat different ontological statuses, about social relations. These were that:

1 Science, including medical science, may be regarded as a 'social' product – its content and practice reflect the social backgrounds and motives of its practitioners, rather than existing in some pure, uncontaminated ahistorical mode.
2 The professional ideologies, status and organization of the medical profession militate against recognition of the universe and impact of the 'social' in health care.
3 The survival and health of mothers and babies is consistently worse in socially disadvantaged than in socially advantaged groups.
4 Differences in social position and experience, especially as mediated by stress, are linked with different fates of mothers

and babies.

5 Social support is good for health.

6 Being researched may in this sense be health-promoting (though it is also the case that being researched may not be experienced as supportive).

These sets of observations derived from my experience of research over a long period of time. Two projects were particularly important. The first was one on women's transition to motherhood (Oakley 1979; Oakley 1980), which led to insights about both the stress-producing character of much modern antenatal 'care' and the extent to which research interviews might be construed as supportive experiences for those 'being researched'. The second area of work concerned perinatal medical issues, specifically a project on the development of antenatal care as a screening programme, in which I learnt how much of modern reproductive care must be called 'unscientific' in the sense that it has not been systematically evaluated and shown to be effective, appropriate and safe (see Oakley 1984; Chalmers *et al.* 1989).

The wider cultural context in which the SSPO project was conceived was also important. Government reports and pressure groups were, at the time, vociferously making some strangely simplistic claims about the state of Britain's perinatal health services. Britain's record of baby deaths was described as a 'holocaust' (Court Report 1976), and 'guestimates' cited 10,000 British babies as dying or being handicapped every year as result of shortfalls in the maternity services (Social Services Committee 1980). Many of the recommendations put forward in the Social Services Committee's Report on Perinatal and Neonatal Mortality and taken up by the media and by pressure groups to correct this state of affairs, pushed for more, and especially more centralized high technology medical care; this was despite lack of evidence that these would be appropriate or effective solutions, and on the shaky assumption that medical care could compensate for or override the health-damaging effects of material disadvantage.

'Social class', 'perinatal mortality' and 'low birth-weight' were key terms in this debate. Britain's record in caring for mothers and babies was widely compared with, and seen to be deficient in relation to, those of other countries, in terms of the narrow indicator of perinatal mortality rates. Behind perinatal mortality rates lurked the importantly culture- and class-differentiated factor of low birth-weight (LBW) babies – babies born too small (weighing less than 2,500 gm) to have a normal chance of survival. Indeed, the condition of low birth-weight babies symbolized much of the debate about the present, future and meaning of the perinatal health services in the 1970s and 1980s: arbitrarily divided from their 'normal' peers by the finer points of hospital scales and official statisticians' calculations, LBW babies appeared ideologically both as exemplar and proof of biology's operation in determining the social (obstetrical) product, and of medicine's parallel rhetoric in claiming – in the pursuit of the 'perfect' baby – to repair or mask all known biological flaws.

The central idea of the SSPO study was to provide and evaluate, by means of a randomized controlled trial, the effectiveness of a social support intervention for women at risk of having a LBW baby. This goal, together with the study's origins, dictated an uneasy epistemological position for the research: one between the two worlds delineated in Table 1.1. The pairs of words shown in Table 1.1 describe a fundamental cultural theme: a dichotomous discourse which inhabits all corners of our culture, including academic work and research funding. The very title of the SSPO study appears to confirm the message of Table 1.1's two models divide: social support *and* pregnancy outcome. The social, the qualitative, the hard-to-measure, is on the one side, the biological, the quantitative, the easy-to-measure on the other. The province of the study was both social and medical; though the intervention to be tried was social in character, the usual health service interventions in the lives of pregnant women are medical. Though an important reason for undertaking the study had to do with social class differences in perinatal health and illness, the denominator population was to be a group defined in terms of a medical indicator – that of birth-weight. The measure of the study's success was to be a mix of social and medical outcomes, from women's satisfaction to use of high technology neonatal care. The evaluation of the intervention depended on use of experimental quantitative methods, but was in itself qualitative.

Designing the study

In my early notes on the study made in 1981, the research design consisted of taking about fifty women with a previous LBW baby and twenty women without, and interviewing each four or five times

Table 1.1 Cultural Dichotomies

Social	Medical
Subjective	Objective
Experience	Knowledge
Observation	Intervention
Qualitative	Quantitative
Practice	Theory
Emotion	Reason
Nature	Culture
Feminine	Masculine
'Soft'	'Hard'
Women	Men
Health	Disease
Care	Control
Private	Public
Community	Institute
Value	Fact

during pregnancy. The focus of the study was to be on stress and life events, but the social circumstances of 'high' and 'low' risk mothers would also be documented. A control group would be taken to provide a measure of the 'Hawthorne effect'. However, my notes show that I quickly moved from this proposal to the design of a randomized controlled trial. Presumably one reason for this shift was conversion by my colleagues in the unit in which I was working – the National Perinatal Epidemiology Unit (NPEU) in Oxford, later famous for its advocacy of randomized controlled trials (RCTs) in perinatal medicine. Another was the intellectual realization that the elegantly simple method of the RCT, together with its logically necessary constituent of some sort of action or intervention 'package' (intended to change something in order better to arrive at an understanding of it) did, indeed, have an unexplored applicability to topics of sociological enquiry.

The second draft design for the study proposed to identify a sample of 200 obstetrically-at-risk women and randomly allocate them either to receive supportive social science interviewing (see Oakley 1981; Finch 1984) or to receive antenatal-care-as-usual. The aim of the interviewing, aside from the provision of social support, was the collection of detailed social data on areas such as nutrition, smoking, work and so forth. The two aims were combined in order to avoid the putting of every available egg into the same basket; in the event of the social support intervention not working, the data collected during it could be used to explore some of the links between social variables during pregnancy and the fate of mother and child. Study 'outcomes' were, as before, to be a combination of the biological – for example birth-weight – and the social – for example mothers' satisfaction with their experiences.

I set about the task of obtaining funding for the SSPO study in late 1981, four months before my current research contract was due to end (it was in fact, and happily, extended for a further year). I first wrote to Raymond Illsley, Professor and Director of the Medical Research Council's Medical Sociology Unit in Aberdeen, long-time researcher on social aspects of reproduction, and Chair of the Social Affairs Committee of the Social Science Research Council (SSRC) asking him to comment on the study outline. A letter in reply said,

> I agree that an approach of the kind you suggest would be valuable. Since our early in-depth studies of first pregnancies in the 1950s there has been no serious attempt to chart the events of pregnancy in a comprehensive fashion taking into account the various parameters of behaviour, nutritional, income and expenditure and psychological influences.

He went on to say that,

> My major reservation applies to the size of the sample. However valuable your descriptive account of the experience of pregnancy, given your initial hypotheses and the design of the study, its potential value will be judged upon (1) its ability to demonstrate an intervention effect; (2) its ability to interpret the meaning of any intervention effect. I do not believe that this can be done using only 100 index and 100 control cases.

As to funding, Illsley observed that,

> the study fits awkwardly (like many good ideas) between MRC and SSRC. My first resort would be DHSS, who are likely to be both informed and sympathetic.

Taking account of Illsley's comments, and in particular increasing the proposed sample size, I redrafted the outline, prefacing it with a fairly extensive review of some of the social factors and pregnancy literature. In January 1982 I sent it out to the eighteen members of the Board of Advisers to the NPEU. Twelve replied, many with detailed comments. In addition, I sent the proposal to a number of other people in this country and abroad including paediatricians, epidemiologists and social scientists.

The comments received at this stage do, I think, throw a good deal of light on the context within which the research came eventually to be done, and which, in important ways, limits the kind of research it is possible to do in this field. Again, we come back to the limits of the cultural discourse represented in Table 1.1.

Two of the three social scientists I consulted felt positive about the study, though each raised important limitations of the proposal as it stood from a social science point of view: the fact that low birth-weight 'is many things', so that its use to define 'risk' mixes different groups, at least some of which will prove not to be 'at risk' at all; the need to understand the *processes* that link social factors and the fate of pregnancy; social variation in medical definitions and terminologies themselves; and possible undercosting of the study in terms of the amount of time the intervention would require. The third social scientist, well known for his work on the aetiology of psychiatric disorder, was sceptical about the notion of an *intervention* study, on the grounds that the precise role of psychosocial factors in pregnancy needed first to be established. A long letter from a representative of one of the maternity services user-organizations raised a different, but very valid, point about the content of the proposed social support, observing that, from the point of view of the study women, practical help with housework and child care was likely to figure prominently under this heading: would the intervention in fact cater for such practical needs?

The more medically-oriented comments ranged from the highly technical to the pessimistically practical. One over-committed medical statistician began his letter with,

> Your draft proposal was put on one side until I had a nice quiet train journey. . . . I have read this with interest, though wonder whether you will be producing a somewhat shorter version before submission – I say this because many referees are extremely busy, not necessarily motivated to read lengthy material, and require it to be presented to them in a way that it is easy to absorb.

Viewing the proposed study within the context of complaints made by women about maternity care, an Australian epidemiologist underlined the importance of considering medical care itself a source of stress in pregnancy. She noted that,

I've come across several women in the past month who didn't come for any antenatal care in the present pregnancy – one because she did last time and still had a stillbirth; the others because they kept being admitted for suspected fetal growth retardation last time (causing enormous family problems each time) – and gave birth to infants of normal weight!

In a similarly realistic vein, from a British community physician, came the comment that:

It seems a most important proposal and I very much hope it can be funded. My experience of medical bodies makes me pessimistic, but perhaps the SSRC might be more hopeful.

'The problem with the research design'

As a result of these comments, the proposal was revised in a number of minor ways before being submitted to the SSRC at the end of April 1982 for a 1 May deadline; the decision would be taken in November. The final decision to send the proposal to the SSRC was taken following informal discussions with the DHSS, who provided core funding for the NPEU, and, after careful consideration, said it would support the proposal to the extent of committing itself to a half-share of the funding. However, the process of sending the proposal out to referees for comment prior to a funding decision was to be left to the SSRC.

The project was costed at over £200,000. The SSRC wrote requesting a detailed breakdown of how many journeys would be made and at what cost per journey. It also informed me that I had to make a strong case for claiming an electric typewriter, and 'as regards the other equipment' (five tape recorders and accessories for the four interviewers and myself to carry out the supportive home interviewing – of which a proportion was to be taped), 'perhaps you could explain how this would be used during the research?' I wrote explaining that the tape recorders were to be used for tape recording, and to provide details of the current scarcity of electric typewriters in the NPEU.

Having sorted out these matters, the SSRC wrote on 29 July saying that it had been decided to hold a site visit for the application 'as is usual with applications of this scale'. The object of this exercise was for SSRC representatives to discuss the proposed research with the applicant, for the applicant to answer any points made anonymously by referees, and then to revise the application before its final consideration by the whole committee. I would be sent an abstract of referees' comments in good time before the site visit, which was eventually scheduled for 7 October. 'Site visit' did, however, turn out to be something of a misnomer, as we were all asked to go to the SSRC office in Temple Avenue, instead of the SSRC representatives coming to see us in Oxford where the research would be located.

A telephone call made in early September to pursue the promised abstract of referees' comments elicited the information that even if the study was funded, it could not start in March 1983 as planned, as there was no money available; 'nothing before June', I wrote despondently in my file, noting that this would leave me salary-less for three months. The abstract arrived three weeks before the site visit. The comments of the SSRC referees were arranged under headings: Research design; Definition of variables; Methodology. Under the first heading came the following remark:

> The problem with the research design is that this particular combination of an essentially quantitative question about repro- duction, 'what is the impact of extra hand holding during pregnancy on final birth-weight' and essentially theoretical con- cerns about the sociology of confinement 'in what ways does social class operate through pregnancy' leads to inappropriate research designs for both.

My notes show that at the site visit I planned to defend myself thus:

> [It] seems to me that *both* questions ideally demand *larger* sample numbers than I have proposed . . . I don't see one objective – the intervention – as quantitative and the other – data-collection on social factors – as theoretical. Both appear to me to demand a *quantitative* approach and to raise important questions about the factors mediating between the environment on the one hand and health and illness on the other, and about the appropriateness (or otherwise) of current patterns of clinical care during pregnancy to this interaction.

The next point was one about sampling – that antenatal care varies between hospitals, and Oxford (which I was not proposing to use in any case) was untypical as it 'has half the national average of perinatal deaths'. To this I responded somewhat sharply by reminding the SSRC that, since randomization would be carried out *within* each centre any differences in antenatal care routines *between* centres should not bias the results. Additionally,

> [The] point about Oxford having a lower than average PMR and a lower incidence of LBW is true, but again this misses the crucial point which is that the recurrence rate of LBW is the same in Oxford as elsewhere. Since the incidence is lower one would expect a smaller number of cases over a specified period of time meeting the criterion for the trial (a previous LBW delivery) but, once included, one would not expect there to be anything untypical about these cases as opposed to those entered from other centres.

The next objection was that the sample would not be representative *because* it was a high risk group, and the special medical care the study women would receive would be likely to invalidate the results of the intervention study. I repeated the argument of the proposal that it was not intended to be a sample representative of all pregnant women, it was supposed to be a sample representative of all women with a history of LBW delivery, and that the reasons for choosing a 'high risk' sample were to maximize the chances of showing an effect of the proposed intervention:

> The grounds for choosing . . . this group [are that it] contributes heavily to the group of babies with the greatest chance of dying in the perinatal period. There are no theoretical grounds for supposing that if the intervention works in this group it will not work in the pregnant population as a whole . . . I think it's worth remembering that even after having two LBW babies a woman has a 70 per cent chance of producing a normal weight baby . . . .
> On the matter of exceptional attitudes and exceptional treatment . . . some hospitals would give extra care to women with this kind of obstetric history, while others may not; however this doesn't really matter from the viewpoint of the research design since random allocation should achieve an equal distribution between experimental and control groups of whatever type of care is practised in any particular centre.

The final comment under this heading was that factors contributing to birth-weight such as maternal height and length of gestation needed to be held equal in the two groups. Again, I reminded the SSRC of the principles of a randomized controlled design; that unless one was very unlucky, the use of random numbers to decide which women were offered the intervention and which were not should secure the same distribution of the short and the tall (and the in-between) in the two groups.

Moving on to 'Sampling' I found myself again confronted with the objection that 'a random sample would not be able to yield details of causes and effects. One possibility might be a matched pairs design of 200 subjects to control for some of the unwanted variables'. I held my breath and refrained from pointing out that no sample ever in itself 'yielded causes and effects', and indeed it was arguable to what extent any social science research ought to framed in these terms. Instead I reiterated the by now boring point that use of an RCT does away with the need to control for 'unwanted' variables – even supposing one has any way of knowing in advance what these might be.

When it came to the section of comments on 'Definition of variables' the referees appeared to be confused by my notion of 'socially supportive interviewing'. Their remarks indicated that they saw interviewing as interviewing and social support as something quite different. They were also concerned about the policy implications – if the intervention proved successful, how could or should antenatal services be reorganized? I replied to the effect that the model of interviewing as merely data collection was based on a fundamental misunderstanding of this aspect of research – on a refusal to see it as a social relationship. To the latter point I responded by commenting that this was essentially a trial of a non-clinical form of antenatal care in an era when most medical routines for pregnancy care were moving in the direction of *more* clinical care and more technology – despite the fact that these had not been shown to be effective, either in general, or in terms of caring for women with poor obstetric histories. This was a main reason for deciding in the end to use research midwives as the providers of social support in the study (under some pressure from the Department of Health which eventually provided funding, and which was also concerned about the policy implications of using social scientists to provide the support). Social care for childbearing women has traditionally been an important part of the midwife's job – and it is what many midwives find themselves increasingly unable to provide in the context of high technology hospital-based care. The first objective, therefore, was to see if the alternative approach of non-clinical, *social* care worked – then to identify why it did, and what should be done about it. These aims could not necessarily all be achieved within the limits of one study.

The next confusion apparent in the comments was between social class and social support: first, that the social class gradient in perinatal outcome would disappear if 'other concomitant factors' were taken into account; second, how would the relative contributions of social class and social support to pregnancy outcome be disentangled? The first comment seemed to me indicative of the tendency to 'reify' social class that is so common in many social science debates. Social class tends to be taken as a 'thing in itself' which explains other things and is qualitatively different from them. (In this context it is possible that social support is a *component* of social class, rather than that the two need to be disentangled.) The second was mystifying, and I replied by saying we would collect descriptive data which would allow us to look at whether social class and patterns of social support were correlated with one another (see Oakley and Rajan 1991).

My responses to the abstract were conveyed round a large table at Temple Avenue to a company of SSRC representatives and delegates, and with the support of three colleagues from the Oxford Unit (Iain Chalmers, Adrian Grant, Alison Macfarlane) and of Margaret Stacey from Warwick University, representing sociology. I recall being very nervous. The outcome of the SSRC's decision was crucial, both for me personally in terms of re-employment, and for a project that had become something of an obsession. I believed in it, and wanted to take it forward. Nothing that anyone had said to me about it had indicated that I was on the wrong track, though most people had (different) sets of reservations. The atmosphere was tense. My memory of the occasion is that within a short time of our arrival, and before our 'external', Meg Stacey, had come, the SSRC announced that it had decided to turn down the project in its present form. However, it was interested in funding me for a short time to work on an alternative proposal. I remember Meg being very angry when she arrived that they had caused her to come all the way from Warwick, having already made the decision. My notes on my responses to the abstract of referees' comment refer to the conversation we had round the table subsequent to this announcement, a conversation which was all rather 'academic' as I was no longer defending a proposal that had any chance of being funded.

The 'site visit' was soon over. Iain, Adrian, Alison, Meg and I repaired to a pub for lunch. We were all in a state of shock, as this outcome had not been expected. Meg and I later went off together to Oxford Street, where I bought a garish red, green, blue and purple outfit in protest.

Explaining to the man in the street

On 22 October I had a conversation with a member of the Social Affairs Committee Secretariat as to the nature of the committee's notion of short-term funding for me. She suggested asking for eighteen months, and had done a preliminary costing which fitted the budget in under a £25,000 ceiling. Would I do a revised costing for the 12 November meeting of the committee? On 29 October I also discussed the situation with Raymond Illsley, who said that the central objection of the 'site visiting' party had been that I needed to specify what social support was first, before undertaking an intervention study to test its effectiveness. I wrote to the SSRC requesting a letter explaining the reasons that the original application had been turned down. There was no reply to this letter, so I wrote again the following January, receiving a reply from another new staff member (the third) saying that he had looked through the file and found 'a synopsis of referees' comments' (the same as had been dispatched before the site visit) which he enclosed, hoping this 'will be of some use'. By this time, the SSRC had agreed to fund me for eighteen months, from 1 July 1983 to 31 December 1984, 'to define and operationalize the concept of "social support", to study the literature, and to carry out the necessary pilot work'. I had been asked (by a fourth new member of the secretariat) to furnish it with yet another revised costing for the eighteen-month period, not exceeding £25,660.

We settled for £27,910, but my attempt to secure in writing the reasons for the original rejection continued. I replied to the fresh copy of the old comments by reminding the SSRC Secretariat that these had formed the basis for the site visit discussion. I went on to say that,

> My understanding (and that of my colleagues) of the discussion that took place on that occasion was that the site visiting party appointed by the Committee agreed that a number of the referees' comments had failed to appreciate the methodology and design of the proposed research. For example [here I listed by number the

comments in question] . . . are not relevant criticisms of a research design that is effectively one of a randomized controlled trial of social support . . . .

It is clearly important that this issue be clarified in the long run if it is my task to produce what is in the eyes of the committee an 'improved' research design. An additional problem is that . . . insofar as the main objective of the 'pilot' funding is to define the nature of social support, this objective is not likely successfully to be achieved within the time period of eighteen months – that is, it will not be possible to answer the question with an experimental design in such a short period of time.

It may well be that in such situations it is normal practice for applicants to be sent synopses of referees' comments only, rather than a documentation of the agreed opinion either of the committee or of the site visiting party. But I hope you will understand my dilemma here.

This correspondence closed with the reply that no further information would be forthcoming:

I can only repeat the problem that was initially mentioned to you, that the concept of 'social support' should be clarified and made operational.

On 18 May I received a circular letter from the SSRC concerning publicity for the pilot project. Would I send it a statement about the project for the next issue of the annual 'Research supported by the SSRC'? It would like 200 words, *'explaining it in simple terms'*:

I emphasize this since it is important that the abstract should be understandable to social scientists in disciplines other than your own, and to the intelligent layman. (This last point has been emphasized by Lord Rothschild, who was asked to review our work recently. A copy of his relevant recommendation is attached for your information. On his authority therefore, I must urge you to suppress unnecessary jargon and neologisms in your abstract.)

The attached recommendation mentioned the most serious weakness of the SSRC as its failure to make known to the general public – 'the man in the street' – its own work and that of the social scientists it finances. 'The efforts of the SSRC in this respect are primitive and unprofessional.' Lord Rothschild took particular objection to the succulent bivalve syndrome ('succulent bivalve' = oyster), and made a number of suggestions about how the SSRC's own language might be improved, including the purchase of four copies of Sir Ernest Gowers's *Plain Words* at a cost of £6.40.

My own attempt at conveying the message of the research to the man in the street went as follows:

Social Factors and Pregnancy Outcome
Social class differences in the birth-weight and survival of babies are a persisting feature of the health care scene in Britain. It is not clear why this is so, despite the fact that the phenomenon has been noted ever since national birth and death statistics began to be collected a century ago. Improved standards and techniques of medical care have not much affected the social class differences, and one reason is that forms of pregnancy care offered to date have not succeeded in lowering one major contributor to the differences – the proportion of low birth-weight babies born.

This study will examine the various explanations and evidence put forward as to why membership of different social groups should be associated with different chances of reproductive 'success'. In particular, it will look at the evidence as to the impact of social networks and supportive relationships (or lack of these) on the health of pregnant women and their babies. Studies describing various kinds of interventions (such as dietary advice and health education) carried out with the goal of improving the chances of successful pregnancy will be analysed. The aim is to design a project in which social support is provided to women at high risk of giving birth to low birth-weight babies, and the effect of this assessed by comparison with a similar group not receiving the social support.

'A change in structure for changing circumstance'?

Some of the lessons of all this are obvious. On a minor practical level, high staff turnover within an organization such as the SSRC/ESRC is an effective barrier to communication both internally and externally. It hardly needs to be said that the fiasco of 'site visits' should not be engaged in when a decision has already been taken not to go ahead with a project. In circumstances where informal decisions are made for shared funding between research councils and government departments, the refereeing process should not be unilateral. And so on. But the SSRC was having a difficult time of its own, and so was social science, and so were the universities. The present tense would do almost as well for all of these statements. There is also an important continuity in the theme of the vulnerability of the contract researcher, who, whilst making a significant contribution to the intellectual and scientific culture of universities, lacks a career status and rewards commensurate with this. A related issue is the problem faced by academic teaching staff, who struggle, for their part, with the nonsense of research 'on the side'. Between 1976 and 1984 contract research employment in English universities increased by 76 per cent; in 1982, when the first proposals for the study described in this chapter were being written, contract researchers made up a quarter of the UK academic work force, and the majority of them were on contracts of less than three years' duration (Advisory Board for the Research Councils 1989).

Bell (1984) and others have told the story of what was happening to the SSRC around the time it was asked to make a decision about the SSPO proposal. It is clear from these accounts that the timing of the proposal could not have been worse. Successive cuts to the SSRC's budget had been announced, and successively smaller proportions of its expenditure had been channelled in the direction of sociological research. By 1976, 91 per cent of the SSRC's expenditure on new research programmes went to work on economic forecasting, organizational decision-making and management, educational management and performance and the analysis of public sector policy (Bell 1984: 20). In the summer of 1981 the University Grants Committee decreed a reduction in social science places in universities; the heyday of British sociology was over, with contraction substituted for the expansionary wave of the 1960s, when twenty-five new chairs in sociology were established in the space of seven years (University Grants Committee 1989). Also in the summer of 1981, the internal restructuring of the SSRC was announced, resulting in the abolition of the old Sociology and Social Administration Committee, and the reforming of the old committee structure into a smaller set of multi-disciplinary committees. At the end of the year, the external survey of the SSRC's structure and activities under the aegis of Lord Rothschild was initiated. The aim of both these moves was supposedly to increase the relevance of social science research to policy, and to discourage theoretical or fundamental research whose policy implications, especially in economic terms, might be either non-existent or unclear (SSRC 1981).

My own meeting with Raymond Illsley at the end of October to
discuss the outcome of the 'site visit' took place two days before
a candle-lit meeting of the Sociology and Social Administration
Committee members at the National Liberal Club in London,
to discuss and protest about the restructuring proposals. (The
reason for the candles was not the avoidance of illumination,
but the power workers' strike.) Lord Rothschild's report, which
surprised many people by recommending salvage of the SSRC,
though not unchanged, was published the month the money for
the pilot study was granted. Despite the defences of Rothschild,
which recommended that the SSRC's budget be maintained in real
terms for three years, Keith Joseph cut £6 million from it in October
1982. The name change to the *Economic* and Social Research Council
was agreed the following year, taking effect on the first working day
of 1984. Douglas Hague, Chairman of Council from October 1983,
insisted that it would have preferred to be known as the Social and
Economic Research Council, but as this would have resulted in the
same acronym as the Science and Engineering Research Council, the
idea had to be dropped. Hague maintained that the change of name

> does not mean the ESRC proposes to increase its support for
> research in economics at the expense of any other group of
> researchers. The fact that funds for research will be short in
> 1984/5 will clearly mean very keen competition for research
> funds, but a balanced research programme remains an important
> objective.
>
> (ESRC Newsletter 51, March 1984: 3)

Such contextual dislocations explain some of the vagaries of treatment the SSPO research proposal received, and some of the internal
readjustments may (as Bell contends) add up to manœuvres which
did succeed in ensuring survival of the SSRC through subsequent
financial and political attacks. But what is more difficult to explain
is why a project that was not discipline-bound but firmly problem-
oriented was not deemed to be 'fundable' research. As the comments
quoted earlier made clear, a significant problem was the study's
province and design, straddling two models of research – the social–
observational–qualitative on the one hand, and the medical–
experimental–qualitative on the other. One important question
raised by this is the extent to which bureaucratic and discipline-
bound funding bodies are able to recognize innovatory research (see
Ditton and Williams 1981).

The basic (and still unmet) challenge would seem to be one of designing such an organization so that it can successfully act as the bastion of defence for a broadly-based and non-discriminatory social science, without at the same time being blinded either by narrow-minded professional imperialism or by short-term political constraints to the need for imaginative fundamental research. The background for this is Britain's poor record of research investment: alone of the major OECD countries it did not increase its expenditure on Research and Development over the period 1981–6, and a major reason for lagging behind other countries is the greater share of the R. & D. budget in the UK devoted to defence spending (Ince 1986; Smith 1988; AUT 1989). The implications of this resource distribution may be far-reaching, and include some of the public health issues raised by the Social Support and Pregnancy Outcome project. It has, for example, been shown that there is a direct and inverse relationship between the proportion of countries' GNPs allocated to arms expenditure on the one hand, and infant mortality rates on the other (Woolhandler and Himmelstein 1985). What is bad for research may be bad for health, not because research is necessarily health-promoting (even for researchers), but because the same impetus that leads governments to formulate research policies and to invest in high quality research, is also likely to generate a commitment to practices which protect the nation's health.

The tendency for social research to act on and transform the social world at the same time as studying it, has always been regarded as one of the main ways in which the 'science' element in 'social science' cannot be regarded as equivalent to that in the natural sciences. Sociologists speak disparagingly of the 'Hawthorne effect' as the best known – and certainly the most frequently quoted – example of this. However, the Hawthorne effect is much more simply a demonstration of the central thesis of sociology: that people are social beings. The workers in the study were responding to the interest shown in them by the researchers. Such findings are witness to the falsity of 'scientism'; which, as Capra (1983) says, has consistently undervalued intuition, emotion, feeling, and direct individual experience as ways of knowing. The undervaluation of these ways of knowing in both the social and natural sciences has gone hand-in-hand with the biomedical model of human beings as physical bodies subject to malfunctioning. Disease is the breakdown of the machine, the doctor's task is repair by physical or chemical means, and the theory underpinning this sees the body as cellular or molecular biology, not as inhabiting the same frame as a psyche, an identity, a social being intimately connected to the social and material world. In aping the natural sciences, sociology thus committed itself to a biologically determinist model of behaviour – and has spent much of its (relatively short) life trying to come to terms with or escape from the inevitable problems this poses.

As authors such as Hartsock (1983), Harding (1986) and Rose (1986) have argued, the masculine domination of science and of society both result in, and are preceded by, profoundly gender-differentiated life experiences. Masculinity itself is attained by resistance to the enclosing structures of everyday domestic life; in reaching for the world 'outside' this, men simultaneously conceive of abstract conceptual experience as preferable to the concrete and demeaning (Hartsock 1983); indeed they must 'have' such a concept first in order to locate themselves within it. The enterprise of science as an 'objective, value-neutral' activity is consequently 'the pre-eminent patriarchal enterprise'. Its theories and data 'tend to legitimate the ideology and power relations of patriarchy' by insisting both that nature exists to save 'mankind' and that scientific inquiry can yield abstract and absolute truths about nature. Such premises make science the 'instrument for "man's" domination of the world' (Harding 1986).

As Harding (1986) has pointed out, a further critical characterization of the scientific enterprise in modern society that follows from the above premises is that it is 'sacred':

> We are told that human understanding is decreased rather than increased by attempting to account for the nature and situation of scientific activity in the ways science recommends accounting for all other social activity. This belief makes science sacred. Perhaps it even removes scientists from the realm of the completely human . . .

It is thus

> taboo to suggest that natural science . . . is . . . a historically varying set of social practices, that a *thoroughgoing* and *scientific* appreciation of sciences requires descriptions and explanations of the regularities and underlying causal tendencies of science's own social practices and beliefs.

If women are largely alienated from science thus defined, then this helps to explain the fondness of women social scientists for methods of studying the social world that are distant from the quantitative, mechanistic and manipulative model of how the natural sciences operate. Even this is not straightforward, however: the geneticist Barbara McClintock's account of how in her work on the cytogenetics of maize she came to see the Neurospora chromosomes provides an alternative version of scientific activity as it 'really' is, which is at odds with the way it is said to be (Keller 1983). Specifically, what is startling about McClintock's account is the importance of the capacity of union between the knower and what is to be known in facilitating the scientist's understanding of the inherent lawfulness of nature. The feeling of union, it is to be noted, is quite compatible with the viewpoint that nature *is* lawful. It is a matter of the *productivity* in terms of law-discovery of empathy as distinct from opposition. The union of social and natural is, in short, as integral to natural, as it is to social, science. All of which suggests that what is required as an end-point as well as a method is an 'integrated understanding of the relationship between the biological and the social' (Rose *et al.* 1984: 10).

The problem, however, is how to arrive at this point without employing the dualistic language of Table 1.1. The account provided in this chapter is only a partial attempt to arrive at the end-point in a way that seeks above all to be *conscious* of the epistemological routes adopted and fixes thus uncovered.

References

Advisory Board for the Research Councils (1989) *Contract Researchers: The Human Resource*, ABRC Science Policy Studies No. 3, Brighton, Sussex: Institute of Manpower.

Association of University Teachers (1989) *The Case for Increased Investment in our Universities*, London: AUT.

Bell C. (1984) 'The SSRC: Restructured and defended', in C. Bell and H. Roberts (eds) *Social Researching: Politics, Problems, Practice*, London: Routledge & Kegan Paul.

Bernstein, B. (1984) 'A note on the position of funded research staff', unpublished paper, London: Institute of Education.

Capra, F. (1983) *The Turning Point*, New York: Bantam Books.

Chalmers, I., Enkin, M., Kierse, M. J. N. C. (eds) (1989) *Effective Care in Pregnancy and Childbirth*, Oxford: Oxford University Press.

Chodorow, N. (1978) *The Reproduction of Mothering*, Berkeley, Calif.: University of California Press.

Court Report (1976) *Fit for the Future: The Report of the Committee on Child Health Services*, London: HMSO.

Ditton, J. and Williams, R. (1981) 'The fundable versus the do-able', unpublished paper, Department of Sociology, University of Glasgow.

Finch, J. (1984) 'It's great to have someone to talk to', in C. Bell and H. Roberts (eds) *Social Researching: Politics, Problems, Practice*, London: Routledge & Kegan Paul.

Harding, S. (1986) *The Science Question in Feminism*, Milton Keynes: Open University Press.

Hartsock, N. (1983) 'The feminist standpoint: Developing the ground from a specifically feminist historical materialism', in S. Harding and M. Hintikka (eds) *Discovering Reality: Feminist Perspectives on Epistemology, Metaphysics, Methodology and Philosophy of Science*, Dordrecht: Reidel Publishing Company.

Ince, M. (1986) 'Science for all', *New Society* 76(1226): 16–17.

Keller, E. F. (1983) *A Feeling for the Organism*, San Francisco: Freeman.

Miller, J. B. (1976) *Toward a New Psychology of Women*, Boston, Mass: Beacon Press.

Oakley, A. (1979) *Becoming a Mother*, Oxford: Martin Robertson.

Oakley, A. (1980) *Women Confined: Towards a Sociology of Childbirth*, Oxford: Martin Robertson.

Oakley, A. (1981) 'Interviewing women: A contradiction in terms?', in H. Roberts (ed.) *Doing Feminist Research*, London: Routledge & Kegan Paul.

Oakley, A. (1984) *The Captured Womb: A History of the Medical Care of Pregnant Women*, London: Blackwells.

Oakley, A. (1989a) 'Smoking in pregnancy: Smokescreen or risk factor? Towards a materialist analysis', *Sociology of Health and Illness* 11(4): 311–35.

Oakley, A. (1989b) 'Who's afraid of the randomised controlled trial? Some dilemmas of the scientific method and "good" research practice', *Women and Health* 15(2): 25–9.

Oakley, A., Rajan, L., Grant, A. (1990) 'Social support and pregnancy outcome: Report of a randomised controlled trial', *British Journal of Obstetrics and Gynaecology* 97: 155–62.

Oakley, A., Rajan, L., Robertson, P. (1990) 'A comparison of different sources of information on pregnancy and childbirth', *Journal of Biosocial Science* 22: 477–87.

Oakley, A. (forthcoming) *Social Support and Motherhood: The Natural History of a Research Project*, Oxford: Basil Blackwell.

Oakley, A. and Rajan, L. (1991) 'Social class and social support: The same or different?', *Sociology* 25(1): 31–59.

Platt, J. (1976) *Realities of Social Research: An Empirical Study of British Sociologists*, London: Sussex University Press.

Rose, H. (1986) 'Women's work: Women's knowledge', in J. Mitchell and A. Oakley (eds) *What is Feminism?* Oxford: Basil Blackwell.

Rose, L., Kamin, L. J., Lewontin, R. C. (1984) *Not in Our Genes*, Harmondsworth: Penguin.

Smith, D. (1987) *The Everyday World as Problematic*, Boston, Mass: Northeastern University Press.

Smith, R. (1988) 'International comparisons of funding and output of research: Bye bye Britain', *British Medical Journal* 286: 409–12.

Social Science Research Council (1981) *A Change in Structure for Changing Circumstance*, London: SSRC.

Social Services Committee (1980) *Second Report from the Social Services Committee: Perinatal and Neonatal Mortality*, London: HMSO.

University Grants Committee (1989) *Report of the Review Committee on Sociology*, London: UGC.

Woolhandler, S. and Himmelstein, D. U. (1985) 'Militarism and mortality: An international analysis of arms spending and infant death rates', *The Lancet* 1(8442): 1375–8.

Chapter 2

Black women's health matters
Putting black women on the research agenda

Jenny Douglas

The aim of this chapter is to review the available literature relating to the experience of health and health services of black women in Britain and to analyse the extent to which it adequately describes and contributes to an understanding of underlying concepts and perceptions of health and illness. Although there is a growing literature on the health experiences of black and minority ethnic women, research studies have been concerned primarily with experiences of maternity services (Homans 1980; Lumb *et al.* 1981; Homans 1982; McFadyan and McVicar 1982; Clarke and Clayton 1983; Larbie 1985; Currer 1986a). Much of the literature describes family organization and cultural practices to do with childbirth and child rearing, where black family patterns are portrayed as deviating from white families.

The main focus is to examine feminist theory and methodology in an attempt to outline the problems in applying them to the experiences, concepts and perceptions of the health of black women. I aim to discuss the complex interrelations between the dimensions of race, class and gender in the lived experiences of black women. Finally, I will address shortcomings in the field of women's health research and will make recommendations concerning the need for further research in this field.

Race and health

Before examining black women's health research specifically, it is useful to outline the approaches which have been adopted in examining the health of black and minority ethnic communities generally. Early papers and research on the health status and health care needs of black and minority ethnic communities in Britain tended to be disease-centred and often attributed health problems to individual behaviour or culture, rather than addressing social and economic factors affecting health and health status (Donovan 1984; Johnson 1984). Most of the epidemiological research was underpinned by a biomedical model and the focus of attention was on illness and diseases affecting black and minority ethnic communities such as the inherited blood disorders, sickle cell disease and thalassaemia (Knox-Macaulay *et al.* 1973; Davis *et al.* 1981); rickets (Goel *et al.* 1976, 1981); tuberculosis (Clarke *et al.* 1979); hypertension, diabetes (Cruickshank *et al.* 1980); mental illness (Littlewood and Lipsedge 1982) and perinatal mortality (Terry *et al.* 1980; Lumb *et al.* 1981). In the case of inherited blood disorders the medical aspects and incidence of them were attended to, in order to manage them satisfactorily, but there was initially little research into the experience of, or support services for, sufferers of sickle cell disease and thalassaemia. In most instances black and minority communities or researchers were not able to contribute to setting the research agenda, and there was little research examining the particular experiences of black and minority ethnic communities.

Furthermore, definitions of ethnicity in much of the early literature are unclear and where comparative epidemiological studies have been conducted populations have been divided into Asian, Afro-Caribbean and African, and white groups. This distinction itself may be artificial as there are many ethnic groups within these rather broad categories. Researchers have attempted to use 'race' as a biological or genetic tool; but although some diseases may have a racial correlation, 'race' is a social construct and has more to do with social structures and relationships based upon power and domination (Phillips and Rathwell 1986).

Early explanations of the prevalence of particular illnesses and diseases were based largely on cultural explanations which did not accurately reflect complex issues determining health status, health experience and health behaviour of black and minority ethnic communities. Anthropological approaches have often divorced culture from social organization or social structure and cultural groups have been perceived as socially homogeneous groups. A meaningful exploration of the health experiences of black and minority ethnic communities in Britain must incorporate an understanding of the relationship of these communities to the social organization of British society, where racial discrimination is central. A black minority culture is often compared to white majority culture in a detrimental way such that its beliefs and values are undervalued; its norms and values are perceived as being deviant or pathological. A particular example here is the diets of black and minority ethnic communities, which were seen initially to be less nutritious than western diets, although current research demonstrates that they are much closer to accepted nutritional guide-lines than many western diets.

For example, the condition of rickets in the Asian population was attributed to poor diets and lack of knowledge of foods rich in Vitamin D, or restrictive cultural practices which prevented women and children from exposing their skin to sunlight. Rickets was prevalent in the white population in Britain during the Second World War and was reduced by fortification of particular foods, for example margarine, with Vitamin D. In Asian populations rickets was perceived to be a problem associated with specific cultural practices whereas in the white population it was seen to be a problem of poverty rather than cultural or nutritional practice or preferences. Sheiham and Quick conclude, in a review of the available literature about why British Asians get rickets, that there is no single factor and that neither diet, exposure to sunlight, nor skin pigmentation can alone provide an explanation. They highlight further issues relating to poverty:

> In looking for further reasons, it is perhaps worth remembering that in the past in Britain, conditions such as rickets have largely been diseases of economic and social deprivation (as they still are in many parts of the world).
>
> (Sheiham and Quick 1982: 20)

There has been a great deal of discussion about the fortification on either a compulsory or voluntary basis of chappati flour. However objections were raised by the DHSS Committee on Medical Aspects of Food Policy (COMA) in a report *Rickets and Osteomalacia* (Department of Health and Social Security 1980). This report suggested that if there were compulsory fortification of chappati flour, some people may receive increased doses of dietary Vitamin D when they were not in need of it. Many groups argued that if a mechanism had been found for fortifying margarine, then this process could have been extended to chappati flour if the government had the will to do so, and accused the DHSS of racism for not intervening more actively.

Many theoretical difficulties arise with the use of cultural explanations in that often they can impose homogeneity on to a group of people and ignore wide variations in religion, ethnicity, class and gender. Pearson underlines this approach, arguing that racist notions of ethnicity and culture are used to uphold the view that problems exist as a 'result of mis-matches between minority and majority cultures which according to the pluralist view, meet on equal terms' (Pearson 1986: 42). She argues that black people and ethnic minorities have always had a second-class image in the health services, firstly as migrant workers and secondly as patients whose different diets, life-styles and religion were causing problems for the established service. Hence culture is perceived to be the problem, rather than the inflexible, ethnocentric service. Black people are seen as having different cultures and it is their culture that denies them equal access to services and opportunities.

A more adequate framework for understanding the health experiences and health status of black and minority ethnic communities is to incorporate into any analysis the dimension of class and socio-economic position. Several studies have concluded that black people occupy a disadvantaged position in British society (for example Brown 1984). Research on social class inequalities (Townsend and Davidson 1982; Whitehead 1987) focuses primarily on social class differentials in illness from data on mortality rates. There is little information linking the economic status of black communities with poor health. Moreover racism and discrimination remain determinants of the social class position of black people and this in turn affects health. However, the effects of culture upon health experience and health behaviour cannot be discounted. It is clear that culture will play a part in determining life-style, dietary practices, health beliefs and health behaviour and will therefore influence the way in which health and illness are perceived as well as responses to ill health. Thus research on the health experiences and health behaviour of black and minority ethnic communities must include an examination of social and economic factors as well as cultural factors.

Black women's health experiences

Research indicates that working-class women and black women are likely to receive less favourable treatment than other groups (Cartwright and O'Brien 1976; Larbie 1985). Black women experience discrimination and racism whether they are Asian or Afro-Caribbean. However the literature examining their health experiences has tended to focus on Asian women (Currer 1986a,

1986b; Homans 1980) and to look particularly at the influence of Asian culture and religion on both concepts of health and experiences of health care. Here, women's experiences of maternity services have been of particular concern and although Currer and Homans were able to use their research to highlight areas where discrimination is structured into the practices of the maternity services, the main emphasis in both studies is an examination of concepts of health in relation to culture.

A great deal of the literature describing the health experiences of black women has tended to focus on family organization and cultural practices in childbirth and child rearing in different communities in an attempt to explain 'bizarre' or unusual practices. Black family patterns are often portrayed as being deviant, compared with white families (see Lawrence 1982; Parmar 1982). Afro-Caribbean families are often portrayed in negative terms as single parent, matriarchal and lacking discipline (Rainwater and Yancy 1967), while Asian families are seen to be patriarchal and rigid (Kahn 1977; Allen 1982; Ballard 1982).

Research studies on the health of Asian women and families have been concerned primarily with perinatal mortality, infant mortality and low birth-weight babies, with a tendency to attribute high perinatal and infant mortality to cultural practices, lack of uptake of antenatal services and diet, rather than to material and economic deprivation (Runnymede Trust and Radical Statistics Group 1980; Lumb *et al.* 1981).

There has been little published research examining the health experiences and perceptions of Afro-Caribbean women specifically. This may be because early research has tended to focus on issues such as the lack of interpreters, female doctors, appropriate diets and translated materials, and these particular lacks have up until recently been seen as having little or no relevance to Afro-Caribbean communities.

Research studies examining the health experiences and health needs of Afro-Caribbean families have focused on child-rearing practices, nutritional disorders, and inherited blood disorders (Martin 1965; Gans 1966; Stroud 1971; Ward *et al.* 1982). Thus Afro-Caribbean women and their experiences and perceptions of health were largely ignored except for some anthropological work by Sheila Kitzinger (Kitzinger 1981).

More recently Donovan (1986) and Thorogood (1988) have examined the health experiences of black women in Britain. Both are white women and may not document accurately or fully understand the experiences of black women. This is not to say that white women cannot do anti-racist research, but that there may be many experiences that black women have which white women cannot understand or empathize with. Jenny Donovan, in *We Don't Buy Sickness, it Just Comes* (1986), very lucidly outlines methodological and theoretical problems encountered by white researchers when attempting to examine the health experiences of black people. However, in her own research she fails to overcome some of the difficulties she describes. In an ethnographic study of the health experiences of black people in London, Donovan outlines the experience of a sample of Afro-Caribbean people and Asian people in relation to health services, and their perceptions of health. Although the research seeks to examine the effect of racism in determining the health of black people, there has been no attempt to examine the part that gender may play, and little attention has been paid to women as unpaid health workers in the family. Donovan concludes that the informants' lives are more patterned by social, economic and political systems and racism than by culture, but does not explore differing perspectives of class and gender within the black population.

The relevance of feminist methodology and research to black women

Many feminists have argued that traditional social science methodologies have excluded women or have portrayed them in sexist ways (Roberts 1981; Graham 1983). This section of the chapter explores the relevance of feminist perspectives and methodologies, as developed by white women, to the experiences of black women. Stanley and Wise (1983) argue that,

1 The central and common belief shared by all feminists is that women are oppressed.
2 The personal is the political, so that by examining power relationships in personal and family life an understanding of social structures and economic systems can be gained.
3 The actuality of a 'feminist consciousness' means that women are more able to understand contradictions present within life and have a double vision of reality.

They further argue that in doing feminist research, the presence of the researcher should be acknowledged and utilized; it affects the research outcome. Oakley (1981) supports this approach and argues that the paradigms of traditional interviewing where the interview is seen as a one-way process; where the interviewer elicits and receives information but does not give it; where interviewees are seen purely as data; and where interviews are seen as having no personal meaning, are contradictory to feminist theory and practice.

It would appear on the face of it that the theoretical perspectives and methodology offered by a feminist approach have equal relevance for black women. I now wish to examine in more detail some of the underlying concepts and assumptions of this approach.

A feminist perspective seeks to examine shared features in the experience of women and starts off from the basic premise that all women are oppressed. Amos and Parmar (1982: 146), in trying to define the oppression of black women, state,

> Racism is not the only oppression a black woman faces. She is also oppressed in class terms, as part of the working class and in gender terms because she is a woman.

They argue further that because of their own racism, white women are unable to understand the experiences of black women who face racism everyday. Furthermore white women fail to understand a number of cultural traditions which exist in black communities and label practices they do not understand as oppressive. Asian women are often perceived as dominated and submissive (Amos and Parmar 1982), while less attention is paid to the experiences of white working-class women and the oppressive practices of white men.

White feminist researchers, however, while recognizing the inadequacies of quantitative research methodologies and social survey techniques developed primarily by white men, fail to address the issue of white women interviewing black women. There is an assumption that the shared experiences uniting women outweigh differences in relation to race and class. None of the white feminist writers exploring women's experience of health have examined the dimension of race in relationship to the interview process between a white researcher and black participant and the power relations which may affect it.

Donovan (1986) and Thorogood (1988) both point to difficulties that could arise in relation to access to black communities but do not go on to explore whether differences in experiences between the white researcher and the black participant has any effect upon the interview process. Furthermore neither researcher considers the effect of the limitations of her own ethnocentrism on an understanding of and adequate representation of black women's experiences. An assumption of much feminist research is that women as interviewers may share common experiences with the women they interview. This is not always the case in relation to black and white women.

Feminist research examining gender inequalities has focused particularly on the private world of the family and has examined the social role of women in the family. Again, much of this research has tended to be Eurocentric and has ascribed particular roles to women within the family. I have described in an earlier section of this chapter the way in which the health of black families has been portrayed in the early literature. It is this portrayal of Afro-Caribbean and Asian family organization that is central to a critique of white feminist perspectives. The underlying assumption of white feminists is that black women's experience of patriarchy and their relationship to the family and work is similar to that of white women.

Hazel Carby (1982) argues that within white feminist theory the family is seen as the central site of women's oppression in contemporary society and that 'the family', 'patriarchy' and 'reproduction' (which are central to feminist theory) are problematic in their application to the lives of black women. She argues that the black family during slavery, colonialism and the present authoritarian state is a site of political and cultural resistance to racism. A further concept inherent in feminist theory is that of 'dependence' and the material organization of the household. Again Carby argues that black women may be more likely to be heads of households, added to which the economic system produces high black male unemployment; hence black women may not be financially dependent upon men. Finally, within the state and increasingly within white feminist theory (Carby 1982; Parmar 1982), the black family has often been constructed as pathological and more oppressive than the western nuclear family structure.

This issue has been examined in relation to health by Currer (1986b) in a study of Pathan women and mental health. She demonstrated that assumptions about the authority of the husbands of Pathan women and purdah were incorrect.

To summarize: white feminist analyses of black families have often been ethnocentric, with little recognition that the internal worlds of black women are very different from those of white women in terms of the relationship of women to work, to the family and to concepts of the family. Furthermore, although there is a complex interrelationship between race, class and gender, for black women racism is paramount (Carby 1982; Parmar 1982; Amos and Parmar 1982).

Feminist theory and methodology fail to incorporate the external factors impinging upon black women as well as internal factors in that the experiences of black women are circumscribed by racism within society. In so far as feminist theory and methodology are products of white society, it can be argued that they too reflect ethnocentrism, individualism and racism and do not allow for the everyday life experiences of black women to be addressed and incorporated.

Developing a research methodology to document and describe black women's experience of health services

There is a dearth of literature which adequately documents and explores the experiences of black women in relation to health and health services. Many policy documents examining the health needs of black communities (Training in Health and Race 1984; Pearson 1985) point to the need to develop health services that are more sensitive to black communities in general and black women in particular, but there is very little documented research identifying specific issues or areas for concern. One of the few published pieces of research by a black woman documenting the health experiences of other black women is a survey of young Afro-Caribbean women's experiences and perceptions of pregnancy and childbirth (Larbie 1985). Another is *The Heart of the Race: Black Women's Lives in Britain* (Bryan *et al.* 1985), in which three black women document the experiences of some black women in relation to health. In a review of research about women who become pregnant early in life, Ann Phoenix argues that narrow cultural definitions are used to explain why young Afro-Caribbean women become pregnant and that this approach masks similarities between black mothers and white mothers (Phoenix 1988). There is a growing body of research and documentation on racial discrimination within the health service in relation to the employment of black health workers (Doyal *et al.* 1980; Baxter 1988). The research on this discrimination focuses primarily on racism and only a few studies have tried to examine the interplay between racism and sexism (Torkington 1984).

The major difficulty in exploring black women's experiences and concepts of health is to find a way to express the complex interrelationships of class, race and gender without being constrained by any one of them. Existing approaches may be too restrictive in that examining social and economic inequalities may reduce and subsume issues of race and gender to class, while white feminist approaches may subsume race and class and approaches examining racial inequalities may largely ignore class and gender and seek to unite people because of their common experience of racism. Hence in many areas of research black women become invisible.

Research into women's health, and the experience of women as paid or unpaid workers as examined by many white feminist researchers (Graham 1983, 1984; Oakley 1979; Roberts 1981), has paid little attention to the particular experiences of black women and has assumed that the experience of all women is predominantly circumscribed by gender. Graham (1991) reviews the way in which the concept of caring has been theorized within British feminist research and argues that research on caring has remained largely untouched by black feminist and anti-racist scholarship. Hence contemporary white feminist analyses do not provide the means either for understanding or challenging the position of black women. Although gender is the main concern in the research on caring, the lack of reference to the experiences of black women as paid or unpaid carers in this area is to suggest that white feminist analysis has been racist in terms of the invisibility of black women.

There are indeed many areas of women's health where the concerns of black women have not been addressed to any great extent. These include the health experiences of older women of the menopause and the mental health experiences of black women. Mental health is a further area where the research that has been conducted has been based upon stereotyped cultural assumptions. Again this approach attempts to impose cultural homogeneity on to a particular group and has made little attempt to examine structural factors. Cultural labels are used as a means of identifying an individual's culture as significant rather than social or material circumstances experienced by black and minority ethnic communities in Britain. Inappropriate terms to describe mental illness have been developed, for example 'West Indian Psychosis' (Rack 1982) and 'Begum Syndrome' (Littlewood and Lipsedge 1982).

Thus to conclude this section, methodologies and theories need to be further developed to take account of the complexities of race, gender, class as well as culture and the relationship of black women to their families and communities and to paid and unpaid work. I have attempted to review the existing research in relation to health and its relevance to black women. Only limited aspects of the lives of black women have been documented and more work is needed to describe wider aspects of their lives in relation to the public and the private domains as well as paid and unpaid labour.

Black women's health: the future

This chapter has sought to identify some of the gaps which exist both in current research about the health needs of black women and the methodological and theoretical frameworks which have been adopted to date. Further research is needed on areas already identified, but also black women must be involved in setting the research agenda and conducting future research. Many academic organizations are structured in such a way that black women are excluded from the research process. Academic institutions presently involved in women's health research need to give consideration to how structures will be developed to allow positive development of work in this field.

References

Allen, S. (1982) 'Perhaps a seventh person?', in C. Husband (ed.) *Race in Britain*, London: Hutchinson.

Amos, V. and Parmar, P. (1982) 'Resistances and responses: The experiences of black girls in Britain', in A. McRobbie and T. McCabe (eds) *Feminism for Girls: An Adventure Story*, London: Routledge & Kegan Paul.

Ballard, R. (1982) 'South Asian families in Britain', in *Families in Britain*, in R. Rapoport and R. Rapoport (eds), London: Routledge & Kegan Paul, 179–204.

Baxter, C. (1988) *The Black Nurse: An Endangered Species*, Cambridge: National Extension College for Training in Health and Race.

Brown, C. (1984) *Black and White Britain*, Third Policy Studies Institute Survey, Aldershot: Gower.

Bryan, B., Dadzie, S., Scafe, S. (1985) *The Heart of the Race: Black Women's Lives in Britain*, London: Virago.

Carby, H. V. (1982) 'White women listen! Black feminism and the boundaries of sisterhood', in Centre for Contemporary Cultural Studies, *The Empire Strikes Back*, London: Hutchinson.

Cartwright, A. and O'Brien, M. (1976) 'Social class variations in health care and in the nature of general practitioner consultations', in M. Stacey (ed.) *The Sociology of the National Health Service*, Sociological Review Monograph 22, Keele: University of Keele.

Clarke, M., Samani, N., Diamond, P. (1979) 'Tuberculosis mortality among immigrants', *Community Medicine* 1: 23–8.

Clarke, M. and Clayton, D. G. (1983) 'Quality of obstetric care provided for

Asian immigrants in Leicestershire', *British Medical Journal* 286: 621–3.

Cruickshank, J. K., Beevers, D. G., Osbourne, V. L. and Haynes, R. (1980) 'Heart attack, stroke, hypertension and diabetes in West Indians, Asians, and Whites in Birmingham, England', *British Medical Journal* 287: 1108.

Currer, C. (1986a) 'Health Concepts and Illness Behaviour: the Case of Pathan Mothers in Britain', Ph.D. thesis, University of Warwick.

Currer, C. (1986b) *The Mental Health of Pathan Mothers in Bradford: A Case Study of Migrant Asian Women*, Coventry: University of Warwick.

Davis, C. R., Huehns, E. R., White, J. M. (1981) 'Survey of sickle cell disease in England and Wales', *British Medical Journal* 283: 1519–21.

Department of Health and Social Security (1980) *Rickets and Osteomalacia*, Report of the Working Party on Fortification of Food with Vitamin D, Committee on Medical Aspects of Food Policy, London: HMSO.

Donovan, J. L. (1984) 'Ethnicity and health', *Social Science and Medicine* 19(7): 663–70.

Donovan, J. L. (1986) *We Don't Buy Sickness, it Just Comes*, Aldershot: Gower.

Doyal, L., Hunt, G., Mellor, J. (1980) *Migrant Workers in the N.H.S.*, A Report to the Social Science Research Council, London: Department of Sociology, Polytechnic of North London.

Gans, B. (1966) in G. Wolstenholme and M. O'Connor (eds) *Immigration: Social and Medical Aspects*, London: Churchill, 85–93.

Goel, K. M., Sweet, E. M., Logan, R. W., Warren, J. M., Arneil, G. C., Shanks, R. A. (1976) 'Florid and sub-clinical rickets among immigrant children in Glasgow', *The Lancet* 1: 1141–5.

Goel, K. M., Campbell, S., Logan, R. W., Sweet, E. M., Attenburrow, A., Arneil, G. C. (1981) 'Reduced prevalence of rickets in Asian children in Glasgow', *The Lancet* 2: 405–7.

Graham, H. (1983) 'Do her answers fit his questions? Women and the survey method', in E. Gamarnikow, D. Morgan, J. Purvis, D. Taylorson (eds) *The Public and the Private*, London: Heinemann.

Graham, H. (1984) *Women, Health and the Family*, Brighton: Wheatsheaf.

Graham, H. (1991) 'The concept of caring in feminist research: The case of domestic service', *Sociology* 25(1): 61–78.

Homans, H. (1980) 'Pregnant in Britain: A sociological approach to Asian and British women's experiences', Ph.D. thesis, University of Warwick.

Homans, H. (1982) 'Pregnancy and birth as "rites of passage" for two groups of women in Britain', in C. P. MacCormack (ed.), *Ethnography of Fertility and Birth*, London: Academic Press.

Johnson, M. R. D. (1984) 'Ethnic minorities and health', *Journal of the Royal College of Physicians of London* 18(4): 228–30.

Kahn, V. S. (1977) 'The Pakistanis: Mirpun villagers at home in Bradford', in J. L. Watson (ed.) *Between Two Cultures*, Oxford: Basil Blackwell.

Kitzinger, S. (1980) 'How the West Indies work', *General Practitioner*, 15 February: 56–9.

Knox-Macaulay, H. H. M., Wetherall, D. J., Clegg, J. D., Pembrey, M. E. (1973) 'Thalassaemia in Britain', *British Medical Journal* 3: 150–5.

Larbie, J. (1985) *Black Women and Maternity Services, A Survey of 30 Young Afro-Caribbean Women's Experiences and Perceptions of Pregnancy and Childbirth*, London: Training in Health and Race.

Lawrence, E. (1982) 'In the abundance of water the fool is thirsty', in Centre for Contemporary Cultural Studies, *The Empire Strikes Back*, London: Hutchinson.

Littlewood, R. and Lipsedge, M. (1982) *Aliens and Alienists*, Harmondsworth: Penguin.

Lumb, K. M., Longden, P. J., Lealman, G. T. (1981) 'A comparative review of Asian and British born maternity patients in Bradford 1974–1978', in *Journal of Epidemiology and Community Health* 35: 106–9.

McFadyen, I. R. and McVicar, J. (eds) (1982) 'Obstetric problems of the Asian community in Britain', A collection of papers from a conference, Royal College of Obstetricians and Gynaecologists, London.

Martin, C. R. (1965) 'Child health among West Indian immigrants', *Medical Officer* 114: 113.

Oakley, A. (1979), *From Here to Maternity: Becoming a Mother*, Harmondsworth: Penguin.

Oakley, A. (1981) 'Interviewing women: A contradiction in terms', in H. Roberts (ed.) *Doing Feminist Research*, London: Routledge & Kegan Paul.

Parmar, P. (1982) 'Gender, race and class: Asian women in resistance', in Centre for Comtemporary Cultural Studies, *The Empire Strikes Back*, London: Hutchinson.

Pearson, M. (1985) *Racial Equality and Good Practice: Maternity Care*, London: Training in Health and Race.

Pearson, M. (1986) 'Racist notions of ethnicity and culture in health education', in S. Rodmell and A. Watt (eds) *Politics of Health Education*, London: Routledge & Kegan Paul.

Phillips, D. and Rathwell, T. (1986) 'Ethnicity and health: Introduction and definitions', in S. Rathwell and D. Phillips (eds) *Health, Race and Ethnicity*, Beckenham: Croom Helm.

Phoenix, A. (1988) 'Narrow definitions of culture: The case of early motherhood', in S. Westwood and P. Bhachu (eds) *Enterprising Women*, London: Routledge & Kegan Paul.

Rack, P. (1982) *Race, Culture and Mental Disorder*, London: Tavistock.

Rainwater, L. and Yancy, W. (1967) *The Moynihan Report*, Cambridge, Mass.: Massachusetts Institute of Technology.

Roberts, H. (1981) *Doing Feminist Research*, London: Routledge & Kegan Paul.

Runnymede Trust and Radical Statistics Race Group (1980) *Britain's Black Population*, London: Heinemann Educational Books.

Sheiham, H. and Quick, A. (1982) *The Rickets Report*, London: Haringey Community Health Council and Community Relations Council.

Stanley, L. and Wise, S. (1983) *Breaking Out: Feminist Consciousness and Feminist Research*, London: Routledge & Kegan Paul.

Stroud, C. E. (1971) 'Nutrition and the immigrant', *British Journal of Hospital Medicine* 5: 629–34.

Terry, P. B., Condie, R. G., Settatree, R. S. (1980) 'Analysis of ethnic differences in perinatal statistics', *British Medical Journal* 281: 1307–8.

Thorogood, N. (1988) 'Health and management of daily life amongst women of Afro-Caribbean origin living in Hackney', Ph.D. thesis, Goldsmith's College, University of London.

Torkington, P. (1984) 'The racist and sexist delivery of the National Health Service: The experience of black women', *Spare Rib* 138: 6–8.

Townsend, P. and Davidson, N. (1982) *Inequalities in Health*, Harmondsworth: Penguin.

Training in Health and Race (1984) *Providing Effective Health Care in a Multiracial Society: A Checklist for Looking at Local Issues*, London: Health Education Council.

Ward, P. S., Drakeford, J. P., Milton, J. and James, J. A. (1982) 'Nutritional rickets in Rastafarian children', *British Medical Journal* 285: 1242–3.

Whitehead, M. (1987) *The Health Divide*, London: Health Education Council.

Chapter 3

Food for thought
Women and nutrition

Margaret Thorogood and Angela Coulter

Since food is basic to human well-being, the role of nutrition in the aetiology and progress of disease should be a primary concern of epidemiology and medical sociology. Food preparation and the communal consumption of food are fundamental building blocks of social cohesion. Women play a central role in both the preparation and the serving of food, and yet much of the published work on the relationship between nutrition and disease has ignored the pivotal role of women. Moreover, epidemiologists have failed to examine the possibility of gender differences in both nutritional intake and disease outcome, often to the extent of excluding female subjects completely from their studies. Much of the published work on the relationship between diet and plasma cholesterol levels, for example, has focused solely on the study of men.

In this chapter we shall draw on our combined experience in nutritional epidemiology and medical sociology to describe some of the different disciplinary approaches which can be employed to explore and illuminate the relationships between food, health and society and we will discuss some of the particular methodological problems encountered in studying food intake. We shall discuss cross-sectional social surveys, methods of measuring nutritional intake, and qualitative sociological studies of dietary habits. We shall look at evidence of sex differences in dietary patterns. We shall also examine the effects of different patterns of food consumption on the health of women and men. We shall argue that the epidemiological and sociological approaches to nutritional topics should not be regarded as mutually exclusive since each approach can illuminate a problem from a different aspect. In such a complex and difficult area of enquiry, as in most areas of health-related research, we believe that inter-disciplinary co-operation is essential.

Approaches to study of diet, disease and the social context of food

Studies of food consumption fall into three main research traditions. First, there are the large-scale cross-sectional social surveys designed to describe in broad terms some aspects of the eating habits in representative samples of the population. The aim of such surveys is not to search for causal relationships between diet and disease, nor are they concerned with measuring the actual nutritional intake of individuals. Rather, they are concerned with describing eating behaviour, such as, for example, whether subjects eat 'health foods', choose particular types of bread, or eat fresh fruit. They use structured questionnaires, usually designed for self-completion, but when resources allow they can also be designed to be administered by a trained interviewer. They usually collect additional data on the respondents' social and material circumstances, and often the dietary questions are only one component of an instrument designed to collect information on a broader range of health-related behaviours. These 'health and life-style surveys' have become popular in recent years as a tool for assessing the health needs of the population, and the potential for change.

Nutritional epidemiology, the second strand of research, seeks to identify dietary aetiologies for disease. Epidemiologists have observed that many of the diseases that are common in western developed countries are extremely rare in the Third World and one of the most plausible explanations for these different disease rates is the differences in diet. There is already a large literature in nutritional epidemiology, though a great many such studies have been disappointing, not least for their failure to acknowledge gender differences. A wide gamut of different and complex methodologies are in use, although, as we shall show, there are still many unresolved methodological problems. Instead of the broad-brush approach of the social surveys, nutritional epidemiologists aim to collect detailed and accurate information about the quantity and frequency of consumption of specific dietary nutrients. Women and men eat a mixture of the macro-nutrients – protein, carbohydrate, and fat – together with micro-nutrients such as vitamins and minerals and the undigested, but important, dietary fibre. For the most part, intake of the macro-nutrients and dietary fibre is much easier to measure, and it is often variation in the proportion of total energy intake contributed by these nutrients and variations in the quantity of dietary fibre which are the focus of attention of nutritional epidemiologists. The intake of some micro-nutrients, which appear in a limited number of foods, can also be measured by epidemiological techniques.

The third type of research which we shall consider is the qualitative sociological studies of dietary habits. Such studies draw on an anthropological tradition to describe food purchase, preparation and consumption in an everyday social context. Qualitative research examines the experience of smaller numbers of people in much greater depth than is possible in a large-scale survey. Using largely unstructured methods of data collection, these studies aim to uncover the meanings underlying everyday behaviour. Such an approach tries to minimize the inevitable distortion of social reality that happens when individual responses are fitted into a predetermined structure. The primary aim of these studies is to develop theoretical explanations of social behaviour.

Sex differences in eating habits

While the family or household is commonly treated by economists as a unit of food consumption, with per capita consumption calculated by simple division from family consumption figures, this is misleading, since distribution of food within the family is not necessarily equitable. It is important therefore to examine nutritional intake separately for men and women (Delphy 1979). However, simply presenting gender differentiated data may lead to the 'gender-blindness' described by Macintyre, whereby differences between men and women are accepted as inevitable and no explanation of the differences is thought to be necessary (Macintyre 1986). In fact, the existence of sex differences in eating habits is a curious social phenomenon which has not received enough detailed attention in either theoretical or empirical work.

In 1985–7 a survey was conducted among a random sample of the adult population in the four counties which form the Oxford Regional Health Authority: Berkshire, Buckinghamshire, Northamptonshire and Oxfordshire (Coulter 1987). A postal survey was sent to 13,000 women and men aged between 18 and 64 years asking about their current patterns of behaviour in relation to exercise, smoking, alcohol consumption, and dietary habits, and about their views on the relative importance of these and other factors which might have an influence on their health. Eighty per cent returned completed questionnaires, giving a large sample which was representative of the population of the region in terms of its social class distribution. Women respondents to the survey were more likely than men to describe their health state as poor, although they reported fewer health-harming behaviours than men: they had lower rates of participation in vigorous exercise and they were more likely to report sleep problems, but they smoked less, and drank less alcohol. They apparently consumed healthier diets, as judged by the significantly greater frequency with which they reported eating certain foods considered 'healthy' according to current accepted nutritional advice (Table 3.1). Men were more likely to report regular consumption of less healthy foods such as biscuits, cakes, puddings and sweets, which were consumed more than four days a week by 41 per cent of the men but only 35 per cent of the women.

Table 3.1 Reported regular consumption of 'healthy' foods in Oxford Region Healthy Life Survey

	Men (n = 5,143)	Women (n = 5,640)
	%	%
green vegetables or salad	70	77
wholemeal or brown bread	34	46
fresh fruit or fruit juice	46	59
skimmed or semi-skimmed milk	26	35
low fat spreads, polyunsaturated margarine	44	49
white meat (e.g. fish or poultry)	11	17

Regular consumption is defined as consumption on more than 4 days per week.
chi-square test on difference between men and women $p < 0.001$

Source: Oxford Region Healthy Life Survey

Women were more likely than the men to agree with the statement that the type of food you eat has a very important effect on your health: 65 per cent of women agreed as against 53 per cent of the men. Women were also more likely than men to indicate that they intended to make changes to their diet: 35 per cent of the women compared to 24 per cent of the men indicated such an intention.

The responses to the questions about dietary habits were combined and a diet score was computed. A healthy diet was characterized as one that was low in saturated fat, high in fibre and low in sugary foods. This arbitrary scoring system does not attempt to represent actual intake of specific nutrients. It is simply a means of combining indicators of 'good' dietary habits to measure the health awareness of people's diets. On this measure, 25 per cent of the men were categorized as eating unhealthy diets, as against only 15 per cent of the women. Table 3.2 shows that the reported prevalence of unhealthy diets was strongly associated not only with gender but also with the social class of the respondents. In each sub-group in Table 3.2 women were less likely to report unhealthy diets than the men.

Similar gender differences in reported food consumption have been found in other studies. In a national sample Blaxter found that women in each age and income group were much more likely to report 'good' diets than men (Blaxter 1990). Women were also more likely than men to mention diet as an important factor affecting health or the risk of illness.

A recent survey carried out by the Social Survey Division of the Office of Population Censuses and Surveys collected data on a week's dietary intake from 2,197 men and women in Britain. There were clear gender differences in the type of foods reported to be consumed,

Table 3.2 Proportion of respondents in the Oxford Region Healthy Life Survey who reported eating an 'unhealthy' diet, by sex, age-group and social class

Age-group	Social class					
	I, II		IIIn, IIIm		IV, V	
	M	F	M	F	M	F
	(n = 1,799)	(n = 1,780)	(n = 2,199)	(n = 2,369)	(n = 808)	(n = 848)
	%	%	%	%	%	%
18–24	24	11	34	20	48	24
25–34	16	9	28	19	39	25
35–44	13	7	24	16	33	19
45–54	16	9	27	15	32	21
55–64	14	10	26	12	38	22

Social class is defined by Registrar-General's classification; married women are classified according to their husband's occupation.

Source: Oxford Region Healthy Life Survey

with a larger proportion of women than men reporting consumption of wholemeal bread, reduced fat milks, salad vegetables and fresh fruit, but also confectionery. Moreover, 35 per cent of women compared with 21 per cent of men did not report any alcohol consumption during the study period and 12 per cent of women compared with just 4 per cent of men reported that they were on a slimming diet during the study period (Gregory *et al.* 1990).

Data collected amongst school children by the Health Education Authority's Schools Health Education Unit at the University of Exeter (Balding 1988) provides some evidence that these gender differences in reported food consumption appear at an early age. Some 18,000 schoolchildren whose schools were participating in a health education project completed a questionnaire which included questions on diet. At the age of 11, for example, 41 per cent of the boys, but just 28 per cent of the girls reported eating chips 'on most days'. Similar differences were observed in a national study of the diet of schoolchildren aged 10 to 11 and 14 to 15, where girls ate more fruit than boys at both ages and the older girls ate less confectionery than the older boys (Wenlock *et al.* 1986).

What is the explanation for these intriguing gender differences in eating habits? They could simply be artefacts caused by the problems of data collection, or they could reflect differences between women and men in the way that they feel compelled to respond to nutritional enquiries. It may be, on the other hand, that they reflect the real situation. If the differences are real, then it is important to explore how it is possible that women and men, who live in the same communities and eat at the same tables, eat differently. Such an exploration could tell us much about the social context in which eating takes place.

Food has a social significance which goes far beyond the mere satisfaction of physiological needs. It has a central place in most celebrations and special occasions. It is used to reward children and to demonstrate affection. It is the focal point of much social interaction. It even has a moral dimension (Atkinson 1983). Attitudes to food can be a marker of cultural differences. Sociological studies have demonstrated a relationship between eating habits and social status which reflect the class divisions in society (Charles and Kerr 1988).

Food has a different significance in the lives of men and women. There are a number of reasons for this difference. Women are overwhelmingly responsible for food purchase and preparation within families. They are also the main guardians of the family's health (Graham 1984). Most education about nutrition and health is aimed at women. Women's magazines are full of advice about food and health. Furthermore, the conventional association of sexual attractiveness with a slim body shape places an additional pressure on women to be conscious of what they eat.

Food is important in men's lives too, but in different ways. From an early age boys are encouraged to eat so that they will grow up 'big and strong'. The expectation that men will have large appetites becomes a token of their masculinity (Newby 1983). There are far fewer pressures on men to alter their body shape in order to increase their attractiveness. Discussion of food and health and slimming diets is restricted to the women's pages. In the patriarchal family which is still the norm, the woman's role as a 'good' wife and mother is closely bound up with expectations surrounding the provision of 'proper' meals for her husband and children (Blaxter and Paterson 1983; Murcott 1983).

The relationship between women and men in the family grouping is powerfully reflected in the allocation of food within the family (Delphy 1979). Women report that men have strong preferences for certain foods which they try to accommodate, often subsuming their own preferences in the process (Charles and Kerr 1988). Women sometimes prepare different food for their husbands from that eaten by the rest of the family (Wilson 1989). Meat, especially red meat, is considered to be a masculine food and is apparently consumed more frequently by boys than by girls, and by men than by women (Charles and Kerr 1988). As we have already noted, men are considered to need greater quantities of food than women. Charles and Kerr's respondents felt that these different physiological needs applied to children as well: boys were seen as requiring more food because of their greater expenditure of energy in active outdoor play. Many of the accounts represent men as more conservative in their tastes, with women often complaining that their husbands rejected new foods and thwarted attempts to introduce a more health-conscious diet (Pill and Parry 1989).

If food has different meanings for men and women, it is entirely possible that the different responses to dietary surveys could be an artefact of the differences in attitudes, rather than an actual difference in eating habits. If women are more aware of current dietary wisdom, they may be more likely to provide 'acceptable' answers to questions about consumption of healthy foods. There is evidence that women are both more knowledgeable about health and disease causation (Farrow, Charny and Lewis 1990) and more likely to emphasize the connection between diet and health (Blaxter 1990). Conversely, it is possible that the different responses to dietary surveys are because women provide more accurate answers than men. For example, if women do the shopping and cooking, one might expect them to know more about the type of milk, or margarine, or cooking fat, used in the home. Men eat more meals outside the home than women (Whichelow 1987; Gregory *et al.* 1990) and it may therefore be more difficult for them to keep an accurate account of what they eat.

Gender differences in both awareness of what is a 'good' diet and knowledge of the particulars of purchasing and preparation of food are just two of the many problems which exist in the measurement of dietary intake.

Problems in the measurement of dietary intake

Variability of dietary intake is a major problem. Few people eat exactly the same things every day, but the degree of variation differs with the particular nutrient components of diet being considered. The total daily intake of energy varies only a little, and it has been calculated that five days of observation will be enough to obtain a fairly good estimate of energy intake (within 10 per cent of the true average intake) whereas it will take ten days of observation to obtain the same accuracy of estimation of total fat intake, and thirty-six days of observation for vitamin C (Bingham 1987). There is also seasonal variation, not only because many foods are seasonal but also because the nutrient content of the same food will vary with the season. It is easy to see that a freshly dug new potato might vary from an old potato, but there are less obvious variations; for example, the retinol content of milk delivered to the doorstep is 26 per cent lower in winter than in summer (Paul and Southgate 1978).

In many cases researchers will be interested in long-term patterns of food consumption. They must then take account of the change in diet over time. An individual's diet may change over time with changes in his or her own circumstances (living with parents, living alone with poor cooking facilities, getting a job which involves a lot of travelling and so on), but there is also gradual change in what the whole nation is eating. These changes can be evident over a relatively short time period. In 1978, the National Food Survey found a yearly mean consumption in the home of 4.44 pints of milk per person per week; by 1988 that had fallen by more than 20 per cent to 3.46 pints. In the same time period, consumption in the home of carcass meat had also fallen by 20 per cent (Household Food Consumption and Expenditure 1978, 1988). Moreover, research has shown that subjects do not remember at all accurately the diet they ate ten or twenty years ago, but, when asked, will tend to report a diet which is much closer to their current diet (Moller-Jensen *et al.* 1984; Rohan and Potter 1984; Thompson *et al.* 1987).

Variation in the diet, then, can be a major problem in assessing nutritional intake. Conversely, for epidemiologists looking for relationships between diet and disease the lack of variation in diets between individuals is a problem. The range of dietary intake within a single population is often very limited, and this may prevent recognition of a relationship which would have been evident if more extreme intakes of a nutrient had been examined. For example, it has been claimed many times, on the basis of nutritional studies, that there is no relationship between dietary intake and blood cholesterol levels within a single population, but when the diets of British people eating a wide range of diets (from vegans to standard meat-eaters) were studied it was possible to demonstrate a strong relationship (Thorogood *et al.* 1990).

When selecting a method of measuring dietary intake it is important to be clear about the type of information that is sought. A dietitian wanting to give advice to an individual with a specific health-related problem will be wanting a different dimension of dietary information about that individual from that required by a researcher who saw the individual as just one of a group, and who was only interested in comparing intake of a particular nutrient in one group with intake in another group. Moreover, for research purposes, it is often the relative ranking of the intake of different groups, rather than the absolute values of their intake, that is of primary importance. This is fortunate, since absolute levels of intake are very difficult to assess accurately. It is much easier to determine that Group A eats more wholemeal bread and wholewheat breakfast cereals than Group B than it is to determine the mean grams of cereal fibre eaten each day in the two groups. (It is important to have some general idea of the levels of intake; it is no good looking for effects of low fibre intake by comparing two groups of people both having mean levels of intake twice as high as that for the British population.)

The choice of method will be affected by which nutrients are of importance. Some nutrients are present in large quantities in a small number of foods, and hardly at all in other foods. For example, 75 per cent of the carotene in the British diet comes from carrots, butter, margarine, tomatoes, and leafy vegetables, that is, about ten food items. Conversely, sodium is present in small quantities in practically all foods.

There are four main ways of measuring dietary intake that are in common use. These are diet histories, twenty-four-hour recall, diet records, and food frequency questionnaires. All of them rely heavily on the active participation and commitment of those whose diet is being studied. They are therefore prone to three major problems: first, the subjects of the research may be unrepresentative of the general population, in that they may be particularly interested in food for some reason, or at least do not feel threatened by an inquiry into what they eat, and for this reason it is particularly important to pay attention to the level of non-response or poor co-operation in dietary surveys. Second, the very fact of being involved in a research study may have made them more conscious of dietary issues and therefore changed their eating habits. Third, what subjects report will be affected by the powerful unconscious significance of food to the subject so that they may report an idealized diet which does not represent the food they actually consume.

Diet histories were the first tool used in nutritional surveys, and date back to studies done in the 1940s. They involve a long interview with each subject. They are expensive and time consuming, are easily affected by interviewer bias, and, moreover, they rely heavily on the accuracy of the subject's memory. For these reasons they are rarely used nowadays in research, although they are still used clinically. The twenty-four-hour recall system also has a long history, but is still in common use, particularly in very large surveys where all that is needed is a snapshot of the average consumption of a large group of people, for example the National Health and Nutrition Examination Study in the United States (Jones et al. 1987). The method is founded on the belief that people can normally recall without difficulty what they ate yesterday and involves recording everything eaten in the 24-hours up to the time of the interview. This method still requires an interviewer to encourage the subject to remember and to record the information; and, because it relies on memory, there can be a problem with under-recording, especially for subjects without established routine eating habits.

The other two methods do not rely on interviewers, but both depend to some extent on the commitment and literacy of the subjects. The diet record method is popular, particularly with researchers for whom nutrition is a primary interest. A diet record consists of some form of diary in which the individual is asked to record everything that is eaten during a defined period of time. The diary record is often supplemented by additional questions about some basic diet habits, such as the nature of the fat used in baking or the number of spoons of sugar taken in coffee. Diet records are liable to interfere with the subject's usual diet. A women with young children who is keeping a diet diary is unlikely to bother to record the half a fish finger and two teaspoons of beans she nibbled while feeding her children at tea-time. She will either not nibble that day, or not record the nibble, and both will be equally problematic for the researcher.

Given the height, weight and age of a woman or man, it is possible to calculate a basal metabolic rate (BMR), which is the amount of energy required daily simply to stay alive (Schofield 1985). (From this formula, the BMR will be greater in adult males than females, and greater in adults under 60 than in older adults.) Provided the energy intake is averaged over at least three days to allow for daily variation, then if the average daily energy intake calculated from a diet record is not at least 1.2 times the BMR then the researcher can be confident that there is some degree of under-recording. Unfortunately, it is not uncommon for diet records to provide calculated energy intakes which fall well below the BMR (Livingstone *et al.* 1990). It cannot be assumed that any such under-recording is random; experience suggests that snack foods and foods with a less 'acceptable' image are more likely to be under-recorded. Another major drawback of diet records is that the process of analysis is slow and complicated. Even a four-day record can involve up to 150 different food items, each of which must be coded for both type of food and quantity. This process can take an experienced coder up to forty-five minutes per record.

Food frequency questionnaires are much easier for both the subject and the researcher. They consist of a check list of foods against which the subjects indicate how often they usually eat each of the foods. Often they have additional questions which serve to refine the quality of the information. They can be self-completed and sent out by post, thus dispensing with the need for an interviewer. They are also quick and easy to code and can even be designed to be machine read. For these reasons they are particularly useful in large surveys. Food frequency questionnaires are particularly appropriate when a nutrient that is present in a limited range of foods is being studied. It is less easy to use a food frequency questionnaire to get a comprehensive picture of the diet, and they are not particularly useful for measuring total calorie intake. It is very important that the questionnaire is tailor-made for the population to be studied, because the foods that make the major contribution to a diet will vary. A questionnaire developed to assess the fat intake of middle-aged women in New England, which might, for example, include questions about sour cream, steaks and seafood, will not be of any great use in assessing the fat intake of schoolchildren in Newcastle, where sour cream, steaks and seafood will not figure largely on the menu.

There is no perfect method for collecting dietary information – all methods have inadequacies, which will vary. In choosing a method the researcher must weigh up the opposing requirements of precision and requirements of convenience (that is, convenience both for the subject and the researcher). The most appropriate method in any given situation will depend on the type of subjects, the type of information required, and the resources available. In all cases, it is essential that the most precise method possible is used, that questionnaires are pre-tested, and that attention is given both to the response rate and to the completeness of the responses. Moreover, information about the basal metabolic rate (as estimated from height and weight) of subjects, as well as basic information such as sex and age of subjects will help both the researcher and her readers to judge the appropriateness and adequacy of the measure of dietary intake that was used.

It is also important to realize that the information that it is possible to collect accurately may be extremely limited in many situations, and some study questions simply cannot be reliably addressed. Recognizing the limits of nutritional research techniques is equally important when planning research and when reading and assessing research findings.

The importance of nutritional research

There is an abundance of official and quasi-official advice on how the population should alter its diet to improve its health, most particularly to reduce the risk of coronary heart disease, but also to reduce the risk of cancer. In order to develop such advice, reliable data from carefully-conducted epidemiological studies are essential.

But these are not sufficient: close examination of the intake of specific dietary components can lead to a partial or reductionist view of eating habits, which is unhelpful when the knowledge thus acquired has to be translated into a strategy for health promotion. Any attempt to change eating habits needs to start from an understanding of the political, economic and social context in which food is produced, purchased, prepared, and consumed, as well as of the social constraints which inhibit change. A social science perspective on the factors influencing what we eat is therefore also essential for the development of effective public health strategies.

As we have seen, women appear to be more aware of the current official line on healthy foods than are men. Nevertheless there appears to be a gap between beliefs about what is healthy and actual eating habits, which is particularly apparent among working-class women (Calnan 1990). This may be explained, at least in part, by the fact that men appear to exercise considerable control over the family diet. Charles and Kerr argue that

> The distribution of food between men and women, and the dominance of men's food preferences within the family's diet, is therefore an outcome of the gender division of labour . . . Indeed, it is a symbolic representation of the subordination of women within the family, a concrete expression of their position as servers and carers of men.
>
> (Charles and Kerr 1988: 83–4)

In the light of this analysis, it is remarkable that there is a dearth of studies of men's attitudes and beliefs about the relationship between diet and health. It seems that both researchers and policy makers have fallen into the trap of assuming that food consumption is a purely domestic issue. Thus both the research and the prevention strategies have been individualized and feminized.

In order to plan more effective health promotion strategies, more attention will have to be paid to the need to illuminate and explain sex differences in eating habits, and to the gender- and class-related influences on food purchasing, preparation and consumption. Women are an easy target for the victim-blaming ideology which pervades much officially sanctioned health education. As others have argued (Sanderson and Winkler 1983; Charles and Kerr 1986; Wilson 1989), a health education strategy which is primarily targeted at women, and fails to consider the economic and social constraints that influence what we eat, is bound to be ineffective. An effective national food policy will need to draw on a more integrated research base.

It is time researchers started to look beyond their narrow disciplinary boundaries. Epidemiologists could reconsider the validity of their methods in the light of the sociological studies on the social significance of food. Sociologists could adopt some of the rigour of the epidemiological approaches to the study of dietary patterns. There is much to be gained by working together to develop a multi-disciplinary approach to this important social problem.

We believe that health promotion policy at present is weakened by a limited understanding of the medical, social and political role of nutrition. Dietary causes of disease can only be tackled by more rigorous research and by greater integration of epidemiology and social science research methods. Practitioners of these disciplines tend to operate in ignorance or mutual suspicion of each other's work. Since there are enormous methodological problems involved in the study of this complex, but crucial, aspect of daily life and health, such disciplinary exclusivity should not be allowed to continue.

References

Atkinson, P. (1983) 'Eating virtue', in A. Murcott (ed.) *The Sociology of Food and Eating*, Aldershot: Gower.

Balding, J. (1988) *Young People in 1987*, Exeter: Health Education Authority Schools Education Unit.

Bingham, S. (1987) 'The dietary assessment of individuals: Methods, accuracy, new techniques and recommendations', *Nutrition Abstracts and Reviews* (series A) 57: 705–42.

Blaxter, M. (1990) *Health and Lifestyles*, London: Routledge.

Blaxter, M. and Paterson, E. (1983) 'The goodness is out of it: The meaning of food to two generations', in A. Murcott (ed.) *The Sociology of Food and Eating*, Aldershot: Gower.

Calnan, M. (1990) 'Food and health: A comparison of beliefs and practices in middle-class and working-class households', in S. Cunningham-Burley, N. McKeganey (eds) *Readings in Medical Sociology*, London: Routledge.

Charles, N. and Kerr, M. (1986) 'Issues of responsibility and control in the feeding of families', in S. Rodmell and A. Watts (eds) *The Politics of Health Education*, London: Routledge & Kegan Paul.

Charles, N. and Kerr, M. (1988) *Women, Food and Families*, Manchester: Manchester University Press.

Coulter, A. (1987) 'Lifestyles and social class: Implications for primary care', *Journal of the Royal College of General Practitioners* 37: 533–6.

Delphy, C. (1979) 'Sharing the same table: Consumption and the family', in C. C. Harris in association with Michael Anderson, Robert Chester, D.H.J. Morgan and Diana Leonard (eds) *The Sociology of the Family: New*

Directions for Britain, Sociological Review Monograph 28, Keele: University of Keele.

Farrow, S., Charny, M, Lewis, P. (1990) 'People's knowledge of health and disease', *Journal of Public Health Medicine* 12: 2–8.

Graham, H. (1984) *Women, Health and the Family*, Brighton: Wheatsheaf.

Gregory, J., Foster, K., Tyler, H., Wiseman, M. (1990) *The Dietary and Nutritional Survey of British Adults*, London: HMSO.

Household Food Consumption and Expenditure: 1978 (1980) (Annual Report of the National Food Survey Committee), London: HMSO.

Household Food Consumption and Expenditure: 1988 (1989) (Annual Report of the National Food Survey Committee), London: HMSO.

Jones, D. Y., Schatzkin, A., Green, S. B. *et al.* (1987) 'Dietary fat and breast cancer in the national health and nutrition examination, Survey 1, epidemiologic follow-up study', *Journal of the National Cancer Institute* 79: 465–71.

Livingstone, M., Prentice, A., Strain, J., Coward, W., Black, A., Barker, M., McKenna, P., Whitehead, R. (1990) 'Accuracy of weighed dietary records in studies of diet and health', *British Medical Journal* 300: 708–12.

Macintyre, S. (1986) 'The patterning of health by social position in contemporary Britain: Directions for sociological research', *Social Science and Medicine* 23: 393–415.

Moller-Jensen, O., Wahrendorf, J., Rosenqvist, A., Gesser, A. (1984) 'The reliability of questionnaire-derived historical dietary information and temporal stability of food habits in individuals', *American Journal of Epidemiology* 120: 281–90.

Murcott, A. (1983) '"It's a pleasure to cook for him": Food, mealtimes and gender in some South Wales households', in E. Gamarnikow, D. Morgan, J. Purvis, D. Taylorson (eds) *The Public and the Private*, London: Heinemann.

Newby, H. (1983) 'Living from hand to mouth: The farmworker, food and agribusiness', in A. Murcott (ed.) *The Sociology of Food and Eating*, Aldershot: Gower.

Paul, A. A., Southgate, D.A.T. (1978) *McCance and Widdowson's 'The Composition of Foods'*, 4th edn., London: HMSO.

Pill, R. and Parry, O. (1989) 'Making changes – women, food and families', *Health Education Journal* 48: 51–4.

Rohan, T. E. and Potter, J. D. (1984) 'Retrospective assessment of dietary intake', *American Journal of Epidemiology* 120: 876–87.

Sanderson, M. and Winkler, J. (1983) 'Strategies for implementing NACNE recommendations', *The Lancet* 2: 1353–4.

Schofield, W. N. (1985) 'Predicting basal metabolic rate, new standards and review of previous work', *Human Nutrition: Clinical Nutrition* 39c, Suppl. 1: 5–41.

Thompson, F. E., Lamphiear, D. E., Metzner, H. L., Hawthorne, V. M., Oh, M. S. (1987) 'Reproducibility of reports of frequency of food use in the Tecumseh diet methodology study', *American Journal of Epidemiology* 125: 658–71.

Thorogood, M., Roe, L., McPherson, K., Mann, J. (1990) 'Dietary intake and plasma lipid levels: Lessons from a study of the diet of health conscious groups', *British Medical Journal* 300: 1297–301.

Wenlock, R. W., Disselduff, M. M., Skinner, R. K., Knight, I. (1986) *The Diets of British Schoolchildren*, London: HMSO.

Whichelow, M. (1987) 'Dietary habits', in B. Cox *et al. The Health and Lifestyle Survey*, London: Health Promotion Research Trust.

Wilson, G. (1989) 'Family food systems, preventive health and dietary change: A policy to increase the health divide', *Journal of Social Policy* 18: 167–85.

Chapter 4

Birth and violence against women
Generating hypotheses from women's accounts of unhappiness after childbirth

Sheila Kitzinger

In any culture those with power to define the meaning of birth also write the script for how it is to be handled and how the different participants should behave. In a technological culture doctors define birth, while women experience it.

Much research on women's attitudes to childbirth defines birth in medical terms, focusing on women as patients, as subordinate members of a hierarchical medical system (Chertok 1969; Day 1982). The implicit goal is to interpret their behaviour for doctors, administrators, midwives and nurses so that patients can more effectively be brought under control, and the system can run smoothly.

But there are other reasons that psychologists and sociologists obtain grants to undertake research into childbirth. In a competitive health care system it pays to take consumer views into consideration. The relationship between providers and recipients of care is increasingly based on a commercial model. Childbearing women are seen as 'consumers'.

According to this model, expectant mothers are offered an array of choices, can select what they prefer, and go away satisfied. This ignores the sales pressure put on them to choose one place of birth or kind of care rather than another, the power of the medical system compared with the relative powerlessness of women having babies, and what amounts to emotional blackmail; this is sometimes practised by a medical system that has taken over responsibility for the production of babies, and tends to treat women as feckless, stupid, egotistical, and dangerous for their babies. Research into women's behaviour as 'consumers' of health care presupposes that they are free agents. As Richards comments, 'Pushing for alternatives in maternity care . . . fails to come to grips with the central issues of who is in control' (Richards 1982).

Research on women's attitudes to birth often also discusses them merely as patients whose lives have no context or meaning other than as patients. They may be recorded as primigravidae or multigravidae, as high risk or low risk, but we learn little about them as women, their hopes and fears, their relationships, and the values that are significant in their lives. Instead, we are presented with scales of anxiety or neuroticism. Women's own accounts of birth are ignored, trivialized or pathologized when they do not match 'objective' facts (Chertok 1969).

The quantitative methods that are usually employed entail enumerating interventions in labour and delivery, rating degrees of dissatisfaction, and recording the length of labour and other physical events. Then the researcher is able to present a series of figures and percentages (Pitt 1968; Paykel 1980; Elliott 1984). In this process the woman's experience tends to disappear entirely. The meanings that these medical acts hold for the woman, the relationship with those caring for her, her sense of self, her body concept in giving birth, and the significance of the birth experience in her life are lost (Oakley 1980; Welburn 1980).

In all cultures the birth of a child is the focus of strongly held values. The behaviour of the woman and of those who assist her at the time of birth and afterwards, together with her initial reactions to motherhood, cannot be understood without an awareness of the meanings that birth and motherhood represent. In western society, this must include understanding of the dissonance that exists between the woman's experience and the culture of the medical system that defines the meaning of childbirth.

In western culture a woman who is distressed after having a baby, who feels that she has been cheated, or that she has failed a vital test of womanhood, is likely to be told that she is suffering from postnatal depression. It is often explained as being due to 'hormone imbalance'. The implication is that the intense and disturbing emotions she is experiencing are all due to her glands, that just as women are unbalanced by their raging hormones at the prospect of menstruation, during menstruation, and also when menstruation stops at the menopause, they are similarly disturbed after childbirth, and that no other cause need be sought. Women are fundamentally flawed (Ballinger 1979; Dalton 1980; Hamilton 1982; O'Hara 1982).

Distress may also be explained in psychoanalytic terms as due to traumatic childhood experiences such as inadequate mothering, some dislocation in emotional development (Deutsch 1945, Bibring 1961, Chertok 1969), or failing these, to expectations of birth or motherhood that are 'unrealistic'. Women set themselves up for unhappiness because they expect too much: 'It is a fairly aggressive, masculine-oriented, non-conservative woman who is most apt to elect "Natural Childbirth". She looks forward not so much to motherhood as to the potency she has always lacked. She is determined to miss not one moment, not one detail of the intensely awaited event, which she fantasises will establish her own psychic virility' (Gittleson 1961: 33 cited in Schearer 1989: 117). In a one-page set of notes on postnatal depression for obstetricians in training Chamberlain states that it is caused by 'unconscious conflicts of the responsibilities of looking after a new baby' which exaggerate pre-existing stress (Chamberlain 1980). Such explanations of unhappiness are based on the assumption that it is the outcome of an individual, internal, psycho-pathological process. The causes of distress are located inside the woman herself, and explained in terms of her faulty functioning.

While the diagnosis of unhappiness as being a result either of endocrinological disturbance or of a personality disorder that can be put right by psychotherapy is comforting for some women, for many others it misses the point. For there are many other causes of unhappiness in women's lives. There is evidence that depression is triggered by stressful economic and social conditions (Brown and Harris 1978). Any mother living in poverty, or who is in council bed and breakfast accommodation where she shares a cooking stove on the landing with several other families, who is socially isolated, or trying to cope with a partner's violence or that of a racially hostile society, is at risk of depression. In short, 'the best predictors for being judged in need of psychiatric care in Britain are to be a working-class mother living in conditions of economic insecurity in a high-rise inner-city flat' (Rose 1990).

There are also many stresses on new mothers, however well-off they are. A baby's inconsolable crying can be a shattering experience (Kitzinger 1990). Even when a baby is 'easy' the whole of life changes when a baby is born. A woman's sense of personal identity and all her relationships are affected in some way. Most women with small children – including those living in comfortable middle-class homes – have times when they feel drained of energy, feel under pressure to meet the demands made on them by others to be good mothers, and are frustrated in meeting their own needs.

'Postnatal depression' is a diagnosis that enables unhappiness to be dismissed as a more or less inevitable part of women's lives, and that 'mystifies the real social and medical factors that lead to mothers' unhappiness' (Oakley 1979). Unhappiness after childbirth stems from a variety of causes, many of which remain unacknowledged. As a result it is either trivialized as a kind of emotional fog that many women must expect to have because there is something inherently unsettling about birth, or diagnosed as a mental illness and treated by means of psychotropic drugs. General practitioners often feel unable to do anything other than prescribe anti-depressants or tranquillizers. Women, in fact, are much more likely than men to be prescribed mood-changing drugs even when they present with the same symptoms as male patients (Hohmann 1989).

What often happens in practice is that a woman's unhappiness is ignored until the point where it interferes with other people's lives. Christine, for example, who suffered a postpartum psychosis, said, 'My husband realised there was something wrong with me when he found me vacuuming in the middle of the night' (Wilkes 1990). When a woman is either obsessional about her household duties or neglects them in a way that disturbs family members, or when she fails to mother appropriately, she is likely to be diagnosed as mentally ill. (Dalton, for example, claims that 'irritability is of chemical origins ... the irritability is reflected on the husband ... he finds that she has changed from the elated, vivacious person she was during pregnancy into the ever moaning bitch of today' (Dalton 1980: 34). Cox defines postnatal depression in terms of a list of symptoms that includes difficulty in coping with household tasks (Cox 1986: 14), and points out that lack of interest in 'preparing food, shopping or working' together with 'lack of libido and interest in sexual activity' can have disastrous effects on the husband (Cox 1989: 329).

Women themselves sometimes believe that a major element in their unhappiness after childbirth is the birth experience itself.

Research into the relation between the kind of labour and delivery a woman has and her subsequent emotional state is inconclusive and the results conflicting. This is not surprising, for it is not simply the number of obstetric events that has occurred, or the length of a labour; rather it is the woman's sense of control over what was done to her, or of being 'out of control', that determine how she recalls the birth, and her emotions afterwards. Women who have felt helpless are at greater risk of postnatal depression (Green *et al.* 1988; Thune-Larsen and Moller-Pedersen 1988).

Though the recording of the length of labour and the number of obstetric events yields manageable numerical material, in terms of the woman's feelings about what happened it is unlikely to reveal any association between the birth experience and her subsequent emotional state. A very short labour can be traumatic, especially if contractions are intense and the baby is ejected like a cork out of a bottle. One in which a woman is isolated from sympathetic human contact, or in which she is processed through a hospital system as if on a factory production line, is distressing even if there are few obstetric interventions. This emerged clearly in earlier research of mine on women's experiences of antenatal, intrapartum and postnatal care in UK hospitals, and led to recommendations from women as to how care might be improved (Kitzinger 1979, 1983).

When a woman has had an operative delivery or a prolonged labour it may, in fact, be easier for her to accept feelings of disappointment and grief about what has occurred. For her emotions are validated by facts which other people acknowledge, too.

Obstetricians may point out that some patients exaggerate negative aspects of labour and delivery. Some tell pregnant patients not to listen to other women's birth accounts for this reason. One obstetric consultant, author of a book for expectant mothers, warned them not to listen to 'wicked women with their malicious, lying tongues' (Bourne 1975: 27). There is often discrepancy between medical accounts of births and women's own accounts of these births. Perhaps such warrior tales of trials endured can be an effective way of dealing emotionally with a traumatic birth experience. But today women are not supposed to tell such tales, and they often feel guilty about expressing anything other than a positive attitude towards the birth because of the effect that it may have on other women who have not yet had their babies.

It is not only this that holds women back from talking about traumatic birth experiences. Many do not believe that their emotional reactions can be validated. They feel that they have no 'right' to the emotions they are experiencing. Moreover, they often think they must be 'making a fuss about nothing'. They are silenced because these emotions are perceived as trivial.

The literature on women's satisfaction with the care they receive in childbirth suggests that they feel more positive if they are given frequent and full explanation and can participate in decision making (Oakley 1980; Kitzinger 1984). When they do not get explanations and are unable to share in decision making they are more likely to feel negative about the whole experience. This holds good at all educational and income levels (Obstetrique '87 1987; Sequin *et al.* 1989).

Childbirth is often stressful. This may be because of pain, medical events and interventions, or, in a complex interaction, stress may result from any combination of these and failure in human relationships.

To label a woman who has been helpless in a situation of overwhelming stress during labour as suffering from 'postpartum depression' turns it into a problem that is located in her disturbed mind, rather than in reality. This deflects attention away from what is wrong with the hospital system and the way that care is given, and from what needs to be changed.

For many women, childbirth is an ordeal in which they are disempowered. Control of their bodies is torn from them. This is most obviously the case with caesarean section. *Cesarean Childbirth*, a report by the US Department of Health and Human Services, lists powerlessness, loss of autonomy and resulting lowered self-esteem as common emotional consequences of the one in four births in the USA that are caesarean sections, many of them unnecessary (Rosen 1981).

It is not only a matter of loss of self-confidence. Women who describe birth experiences in which they have been disempowered often feel that they have been violated. They use the language of rape.

With two of my daughters, Polly Kitzinger and Jenny Kitzinger, who work with women who have been raped, I explored the language that women use when describing their experiences of sexual violence, and compared this with that used by 345 women who described traumatic birth experiences in which they had been robbed of control over their own bodies, and in all of which they used the words 'rape', 'abuse', 'assault' or 'violence' to describe their experiences.

The material in the following pages is drawn from these women's accounts of distressing birth experiences: labours which were not only difficult, but which they described in terms of rape, and in which they felt that they had been disempowered. These were written between October 1987 and October 1989. They include 172 letters that followed an article on the negative aspects of some birth experiences that I wrote for the British national newspaper *The Independent*, and 97 following a television programme during which I referred to the subject. The other 76 accounts came from readers of my books about childbirth. Discourse analysis provided a framework for disclosing some common factors in these accounts.

These accounts come from a self-selected group of women who wrote because they felt strongly about the subject. Their experiences cannot be transposed to childbearing women in general. Yet they may provide clues to elements in childbirth which other women, too, find distressing, and which may affect their postnatal emotional state. I do not claim to prove or disprove a theory, or to be able to produce solutions, but am trying instead to generate hypotheses which other researchers might then investigate and develop.

Sometimes it was obvious that a birth was distressing because the baby died, as with one woman who delivered stillborn twins at 24 weeks. Yet she said the experience was made much worse because 'It was like a rape. Nobody took into account my feelings and I never had a chance to talk about it.'

A typical account came from a woman who wrote, 'This is the first chance I've had to tell anybody the whole story of my ghastly birth experience one year ago.' She described a labour in which she was bewildered by the number and variety of staff attending and observing her, and by frequent disruptive shift changes. Her membranes were artificially ruptured and a scalp monitor introduced without her consent, and with no warning. Then a midwife told her husband to go home. She tried to cope with a rapidly escalating labour without any personal support, and the bell was out of reach. After she had shouted for ten minutes, someone came in and asked, 'What's all the noise for?' Because she had been given an epidural (which was ineffective in relieving pain) she was told, 'It's all your imagination!' Then she said she was suddenly surrounded by people shouting at her to push. 'I just wanted to scream, "will you fuck off and let me have my baby in peace?".' After a violent delivery, her vaginal and perineal lacerations were sutured painfully by a doctor who did not speak to her. The sutures became infected and it was twelve weeks before the wounds closed. 'I was very depressed about everything, kept reliving the birth and thinking, "What did I do wrong?". I felt nothing for the baby, just looked after her through a sense of duty. It was as though I'd been given some other woman's child to look after.' She said she was starting to love her child, but still had nightmares about the birth.

Given an account like this it is tempting to look back nostalgically, and to romanticize childbirth in the past. Many of these home births were peaceful, satisfying and safe. Yet others left bitter memories of incompetence and cruelty, and women now in their sixties and seventies can still describe their suffering in minute and vivid detail. Women have sometimes written to me, forty or fifty years after the event, trying to exorcise horrific birth experiences. One woman delivered a breech baby with extended legs at home, for example, after a labour of thirty hours, and was not allowed to take gas and air. When she cried out, she was told by the midwife, 'Shut up! the men are coming down the road on their way home for lunch'. . . . 'The doctor pulled out a leg [and broke it]. The baby then came out so far, but the head wouldn't come, so my husband was sent about two miles [on his bike] for a doctor with anaesthetic.'

Yet modern technology has increased the opportunities for intervention in childbirth and for rendering women powerless. Birth has been removed from the home to the public arena of the hospital delivery room. A woman may be tethered to machines, surrounded by strangers and so feel treated primarily as a reproductive mechanism.

Many of the labours described in these women's accounts were managed with high technology. Women had tubes, catheters and electronic equipment attached to them. Two-thirds of the accounts describe induction. A high proportion had forceps deliveries or caesarean sections. These often seem to have been the result of a cascade of intervention which started with induction because the woman was past her expected date of delivery.

Induction of labour tends to make birth more painful and distressing. A study of women's experiences of induction showed that those who were induced received larger amounts of analgesic drugs than those who started labour spontaneously. Women who have already experienced a labour that started spontaneously usually compare an induced labour unfavourably with the previous birth (Kitzinger 1975).

In some hospitals augmentation of labour is the norm and women have an intravenous drip set up and an electrode attached to the baby's head. Invasive technology combined with physical immobilization and depersonalization can lead to fear, pain and distress.

One vivid account, in this case of a ventouse delivery, was written in the form of a poem:

He dragged you from me. The surgeon:
His pink head shone under sparse wet hair
An angry face down there beyond my thighs.
Machinery, a massive light, men around you and me . . .
A row of frightened students lined against the wall
Framed by my aching legs strapped tight.
The balding pink man showed them the scissors
And cut me . . .
Relax, he shouted.
He fixed a round black rubber cup to your head,
It sucked onto your head, your soft and furry head.
With both hands he gripped the pipe attached to it
A foot braced on the table before you, he pulled
Again, Again, Relax Woman. The sweat ran in his eyes
And grey veins pulsed in his temples, grim.
Suddenly he took you from me.
Our blood splashed and squirted, scarlet on the ceiling,
The butcher had blood in his eyes.

Yet it was not only when birth entailed surgery that a woman felt violated. Many of these births appear to have been obstetrically straightforward, and the interventions were routine practices that occur in many hospital labours, such as artificial rupture of the membranes, electronic fetal monitoring, forced pushing and episiotomy.

A woman who had 'a normal delivery' like this (no forceps, no caesarean, a live, healthy baby) felt that unlike the death of the child's father during the pregnancy, 'it couldn't be *shared* with anyone, even close friends. I just didn't have the words to explain why I felt so violated.'

In each of these birth accounts women used metaphors of rape. One woman wrote that she could not understand why she was in 'incredible' vaginal and perineal pain after a caesarian section. No one would answer her questions. After three letters to the hospital in an attempt to find out, she was told that 'the baby was so stuck in my pelvis that they'd put my legs in stirrups and entered me vaginally, apparently with some force, to unstick the baby's head . . . I was cut, torn, had a fist in me and was stitched up vaginally without getting to know about it.' When she asked why she had not been told, the reply was that it 'was normal in those circumstances not to tell the woman and wasn't considered important that she should know.' She went on to say,

'I feel invaded and mutilated . . . I don't feel the same person any more.'

Many women described the depersonalization they experienced when among strangers who seemed to be concerned only with the lower end of their bodies, who observed, manipulated, poked and prodded them, and finally cut their genitals. The common thread running through all these accounts is that women felt completely powerless.

It should be emphasized that this was not merely a question of pain. For some women pain was well-controlled, but the birth was still distressing. A woman who was disorientated with pethidine wrote, 'When I came round, my waters had been broken, plus two catheters inserted. The room was full of strangers.' She said that staff conducting the birth ignored her, and she felt that the experience had been taken from her. Another woman was told that she must have an epidural: 'My husband thought it was great because he didn't have to watch me in pain. A lasting memory is of the registrar saying, as he stitched me up, "painless childbirth – it's what every woman wants!" I was too washed up emotionally to tell him that this wasn't how I felt.' Subsequently she became deeply depressed: 'I have been told that it was due to hormones, that I have a lovely baby and should be grateful, that I should be glad that I didn't have a caesarean, that I should snap out of it and stop feeling story for myself, and that it was my own fault for expecting too much.'

The major themes which emerged from analysis of the accounts revealed a similarity between the experience of rape and of powerlessness in childbirth in the following ways.

After birth, as after rape, a woman may suffer acute physical pain and genital mutilation, her vagina and perineum torn or incised – scissors, rather than by a broken bottle or a knife (Kitzinger 1984). Women said: 'My inside is a mess'; 'It is a pulp'; 'I am torn to ribbons'; 'I can never be the same again'. When infection follows, healing is incomplete or scar tissue forms, a woman may be left permanently damaged.

Whether or not a woman suffers physical injury, she is emotionally injured, by being robbed of a sense of personal identity. The rape victim says, 'It could have been *anyone* so long as it was a female body.' After childbirth a woman said, 'He never even looked at the top half of me. I wasn't a person any more. I was just a number' [or 'a case']; 'They didn't speak *to* me, only *about* me.' One woman wrote of her forceps delivery, 'It was as though I was not there.' Women described strangers milling around them during delivery. As one woman put it, 'It was as if I had to put on a show for them . . . It was like a circus.'

Emotional blackmail is employed to obtain compliance by the patient or victim, and she may be cajoled or tricked into submission. In childbirth she may be warned that she must accept hospital protocols and obstetric decisions for the baby's sake. By threatening her with the baby's death, obstetric power is legitimized. A woman described how, when she asked for a home birth, the doctor said, 'You don't want to hurt the baby, do you? . . . It would be a pity to have gone through nine months and then kill it.' In the thirty-eighth week of a normal pregnancy, a 18-year-old was told by an obstetrician, 'I'm not 100 per cent happy with your weight gain.' He told her to come in for another scan, decided that the baby was small for dates, and induced labour. After hours of pain, with 'doctors directing a birth where I was merely a vessel with my contents to be offloaded', a baby of nearly 4 kg was delivered by emergency caesarean section. 'I left hospital with a baby girl I didn't feel I had given birth to,' she told me, 'a red wound across my abdomen, and a lot of unhappiness to follow.'

In childbirth, as in rape, a woman may be stripped, forcibly exposed, her legs splayed and tethered, and her sexual organs put on display to all comers. One woman described how a window cleaner, clinging outside the pane of the hospital window, watched, fascinated, as she pushed her baby out. The woman's body is fragmented, attention centred on the space between her legs. It is as if she does not exist as person – only her genitals. In the second stage it is common to see assistants crowding at the lower end of the woman's body, anxiously watching her vulva as if waiting for luggage to appear on an airport carousel.

Rape and birth trauma survivors are both at first shocked, numb and emotionally anaesthetized. Their dominant feeling is one of relief that they have survived. They long to 'get back to normal'. They try to behave as though nothing distressing has occurred. With rape a woman – even one whose vagina has been lacerated and who is bleeding heavily – may get up and make coffee and chat with the rapist, enacting a ritual, a domestic task, which symbolizes a return to normality. After birth, a woman may try to act the part of a happy mother with her new baby, and say how wonderful her doctor is. This is one reason why patient response rates to questionnaires conducted in the immediate postpartum period are often high, and why women express satisfaction with the care received at that stage, who several months later may express very different emotions.

After a distressing birth, as after rape, women often described what they had been through as butchery. One said the obstetrician 'hauled me around like a slab of meat'. Others felt 'skewered', 'trussed up like an oven-ready turkey', like 'a fish on a slab' or 'a carcass'. It is the language of pornography. They were forcibly exposed and stripped naked, not only physically but mentally. It was as if the inside had been turned out and they were raw and excoriated.

Both groups use the language of dirt and waste disposal too: 'trash', 'rubbish', 'shit', 'a bloody mess'. A rape survivor told how the man urinated on her. Another said of a gang rape, 'They used me like a public lavatory.' After a distressing birth women may talk about their feelings of helplessness and self-disgust, when they were unable to control bladder, bowels or leaking amniotic fluid.

Yet often, too, women can find no words in which to describe what happened. After childbirth everything may be 'explained' in medical terms – and the woman is silenced. It is similar with rape. A teenager sexually abused by her schoolteacher said, 'All the words I had were the words *he* gave me. *He* called it "love".' Women often have no legitimate way of describing personal experiences except in the terminology of the oppressor.

A woman who has just had a baby usually feels grateful to those who attended her. When she has been abused, this gratitude is mixed with horror at the violence used against her by the very people who have 'given' her the baby. She is torn by emotional conflict. In one woman's words,
'The professional team was very efficient. The baby is lovely. But I don't feel a whole person. How long will it be before I stop feeling guilty and cheated? I'm crying now. I know I'm being silly.'

Both rape and birth survivors blame themselves for what has occurred: 'If only I hadn't walked home alone'; 'If only I'd pushed harder'. They often believe they deserved it because there is something wrong with them: 'It was really all my fault'; 'I asked for it. I shouldn't have walked across the common that night'; 'I was a little flirt; Daddy couldn't help it'; 'I'm responsible for breaking up a happy family'; 'I shouldn't have missed any of the childbirth classes'; 'I ought to have practised my breathing more.'

Other people contribute to this sense of guilt. Judges may pronounce the rape survivor guilty of 'contributory negligence' because she wore a short skirt or hitch-hiked. Obstetricians – even midwives occasionally – may do the same. Women were told that they had an episiotomy because they did not relax or did not 'try' hard enough. Several women were told by anaesthetists that it was their fault that an epidural worked only on one side, because they were 'too fat'. Care-givers also told women, 'You read too many books'; 'made that ridiculous birth plan'; 'had unrealistic expectations'.

Many women who have experienced violence in childbirth never make an official complaint. Similarly, of those who contacted the London Rape Crisis Centre, at least 75 per cent have not reported the crime to the police (London Rape Crisis Centre 1984). This is often because, as one rape survivor said, 'I couldn't speak. When I tried to it was like it was happening all over again. I couldn't open my mouth', or because, as another said, 'no one would believe me, and I'd end up being put away somewhere'. Neither of these women told anyone they had been raped till some years later.

Complaining about hospital care can be just as daunting as reporting rape. Women often do not think a complaint is justified because 'the staff were all so busy and overworked' or 'I was so bewildered and dazed by the horror of it all that I didn't really *think* to complain', and 'it was only after a year that I realised the enormity of the ordeal'. The woman who said this had her baby in a military hospital, and after failed induction at thirty-seven weeks had a caesarean section with an epidural, which went beyond the dural space into her spine. This, according to medical records made at the time, produced respiratory and cardiac arrest. She was resuscitated, intubated and ventilated. It was, she told me, 'the most frightening four hours of my life. I experienced a sense of near death. I was terrified that the doctors would declare me dead and that I could not do anything about it.' She had a shattering headache, neckache and backache for several days after and it was two days before she even saw her baby. She made an appointment to try and find out exactly what had happened. The senior obstetrician – who was not present during the birth – told her that she could not have had cardiac arrest, and deleted it from the records in front of her. No one will ever know exactly what was done to this woman. Her husband is in the forces and the doctor is his superior officer. She told me that she cannot take it further because it might harm his career, and it is the only hospital in the area to which her child could go if he were ill.

Grieving after experiences like these is often unacknowledged, or is strenuously denied because women become very isolated. They feel abnormal, 'unnatural', no longer 'whole', different from other women, and different from everybody because of the stigma of their experience. They may be unable to let anyone touch them sexually, or even with affection, and try to protect themselves by keeping other people at a distance. They say things like: 'I don't want to upset other people by talking about it'; 'It's not the kind of bombshell you drop into ordinary conversation.' A woman often feels that she cannot talk to other new mothers, those who were in her antenatal class, for example, because she is the only one who has been through this experience, and must be abnormal, 'and everyone says I'm stupid when I say how I feel'. Rape survivors feel similarly isolated, abnormal and stigmatized.

There are also specific parallels between the experiences of survivors of child sexual abuse and of violence in childbirth. A survivor of sexual abuse said, 'I have been robbed of my childhood.' A woman who survived a distressing birth also felt robbed of a positive experience. She felt cheated. Trust had been betrayed. The woman whose father called her his 'little princess' had been violated by him. The one whose doctor was a sugar-daddy during her pregnancy and said 'you can have your baby any way you like', was betrayed by someone who took on the role of a loving father. When a girl resists rape the father often becomes abusive and calls her 'slut' and 'whore'. He tells her she is selfish for not wanting sex with him. In the same way, when a woman resists an invasive obstetric procedure she may also be accused of being 'selfish', concerned only with her own emotions, and of not caring whether she kills her baby.

Those trying to help a woman who is distressed after childbirth or following rape often want to calm her down. When a woman had almost died from obstetric anaesthesia, she said, 'There was this air of "it never really happened"'. Rape survivors often say, 'It was as if they'd forgotten I'd ever told them about it'. Friends tell them, 'Soonest forgotten, soonest mended'; 'You must put things in perspective', even 'Count your blessings'!

Both birth and rape survivors may be offered mood-changing drugs to calm them. While tranquillizers may help a woman to act more normally, they do not address what is for her the main issue, that she has been disempowered and abused.

Survivors often feel that they should be coping better: 'It's a year and I ought to be over it by now, but I'm still having terrible dreams.' Their anger is turned in on themselves as depression. Hallucinations, nightmares, panic attacks, the way *their* view of reality seems different from everyone else's, makes them feel they are disintegrating mentally. Obstetric management that is invasive and controlling is not unique and special, but is part of widespread male violence against women. The introduction of high technology, electronic ways of monitoring and controlling women's bodies, increases this potential for violence. In Britain 87 per cent of consultants in obstetrics and gynaecology are men. Women doctors often conform to the system because it is the only way to get ahead in their careers, or because they feel helpless at doing anything to change it. Birth in western society has become an institutionalized act of violence against women, and postnatal depression is often grief that follows helplessness in the face of that violence.

Rape crisis counsellors throw a life-line to women who have suffered sexual violence. Counsellors are known by their first names and have resisted becoming professionalized. They help women who desperately want to talk to others who will listen and believe them. There is need for sensitive counselling after distressing birth experiences, too. This should come from outside the medical system. One outcome of this preliminary research has been the setting up of a Birth Crisis Network.

From whatever backgrounds birth crisis counsellors come – childbirth education, midwifery, psychology, psychotherapy or nursing – we offer help simply as women, not as agents of a professional system. Birth crisis counsellors *need* to be free of the medical system because we are also advocates for women – supporting them in making a complaint when that is what they want to do, questioning policies and practices, finding out what really happened, and working towards changing the system. Our aim is to help the survivor slot together different aspects of her experience as if they were pieces of a jigsaw in order to make a whole picture which has meaning for her. She knows that there is someone who will listen and believe what she says. This is how healing starts.

The knowledge that what a woman feels is accepted by others – that it is validated, the realization that there is someone on her side who is prepared to speak out *with* her – may enable her to find strength within herself.

Rape is endemic in our society. The western way of birth proves often to be another form of institutionalized violence against women.

There is need for research focused on women's experiences in which women themselves define the meaning of birth and what it is to be a mother in the context of their own lives and their own values; a need for research not only *on* women but *for* women (Klein 1983; Nicolson 1986). The challenge is to explore women's experiences of childbirth and motherhood in a way that is not trapped in a medical context, and as a result of what is learned about these experiences to work towards creating an environment for birth in which women can be empowered through birth-giving.

References

Ballinger, B. (1979) 'Emotional disturbance following childbirth', *Psychological Medicine* 9: 293–300.

Bibring, B. L. (1961) 'A study of the psychological processes in pregnancy and the earliest mother–child relationship', *The Psychoanalytic Study of the Child* 16: 9–72.

Brown, G. and Harris, T. (1978) *Social Origins of Depression*, London: Tavistock.

Bourne, G. (1975) *Pregnancy*, London: Pan.

Chamberlain, G. (1980) *Lecture Notes on Obstetrics*, 4th edn, Oxford: Basil Blackwell.

Chertok, L. (1969) *Motherhood and Personality*, London: Tavistock.

Cox, J. L. (1986) *Postnatal Depression: A Guide for Health Professionals*,

Edinburgh: Churchill Livingstone.

Cox, J. L. (1989) 'Can postnatal depression be treated?', *Midwife, Health Visitor and Community Nurse* 258: 326–7.

Dalton, K. (1980) *Depression after Childbirth*, Oxford: Oxford University Press.

Day, S. (1982) 'Is obstetric technology depressing?', *Radical Science Journal* 12: 17–45.

Deutsch, H. (1945) *The Psychology of Women*, Vol. II: *Motherhood*, New York: Grune & Stratton.

Elliott, S. (1984) 'Relationship between obstetric outcome and psychological measures in pregnancy and the postnatal year', *Journal of Reproduction and Infant Psychology*, 2: 18–32.

Gittleson, N. (1961) 'The case against natural childbirth', *Harpers Bazaar*, February.

Green, J. M., Coupland, V. A., Kitzinger, J. V. (1988) *Great Expectations: A Prospective Study of Women's Expectations and Experiences of Childbirth* Cambridge: Child Care and Development Group.

Hamilton, J. (1982) 'The identity of post-partum psychosis', in I. Brockington and R. Kumar (eds) *Motherhood and Mental Illness*, London: Academic Press.

Hohmann, A. A. (1989) 'Gender bias in psychotrophic drug prescribing in primary care', *Medical Care* 27: 478–90.

Kitzinger, S. (1975) *Some Mothers' Experiences of Induced Labour*, London: National Childbirth Trust.

Kitzinger, S. (1979) *The Good Birth Guide*, London: Fontana; (1983) *The New Good Birth Guide*, Harmondsworth: Penguin.

Kitzinger, S. (1984) *Some Women's Experiences of Episiotomy*, London: National Childbirth Trust.

Kitzinger, S. (1987) *Some Women's Experiences of Epidurals*, London: National Childbirth Trust.

Kitzinger, S. (1990) *The Crying Baby*, Harmondsworth: Penguin.

Klein, R. D. (1983) 'Thoughts about feminist methodology', *Theories of Women's Studies*, in G. Bowles and R. D. Klein (eds) London: Routledge.

London Rape Crisis Centre (1984) *Sexual Violence: The Reality for Women*, London: The Women's Press.

Nicolson, P. (1986) 'Developing a feminist approach to depression following childbirth', in S. Wilkinson (ed.) *Feminist Social Psychology*, Milton Keynes: Open University Press.

O'Hara, M. W. (1982) 'Predicting depressing symptomatology: Cognitive behavioural models and postpartum depression', *Journal of Abnormal Psychology* 91: 457–61.

Oakley, A. (1979) 'The baby blues', *New Society*, 48(861): 11–13.

Oakley, A. (1980) *Women Confined: Towards a Sociology of Childbirth*, Oxford: Martin Robertson.

Obstetrique '87 (1987) *Canadian Medical Association Journal* Supplement 136: 1–31.

Paykel, E. S. (1980) 'Life events and social support in puerperal depression', *British Journal of Psychology* 136: 339–46.

Pitt, B. (1968) '"Atypical" depression following childbirth', *British Journal of Psychiatry* 114: 1325–35.

Richards, M. (1982) 'The trouble with "choice" in childbirth', *Birth* 9: 253–60.

Rose, S. (1990) 'Mind bending realities', *Sunday Correspondent*, 29 July.

Rosen, M. G. (1981) *Cesarean Childbirth: Report of a Consensus Development Conference* (NIH publication no. 82–2067), Bethesda, Md.: National Institute of Health.

Schearer, M. (1989) 'Maternity patients movements in the United States 1920–1980', in I. Chalmers, M. Enkin, M. Keirse (eds) *Effective Care in Pregnancy and Childbirth*, Oxford: Oxford University Press.

Sequin, L. Therrien, R. Champagne, F. and Labour, D. E. (1989) 'Components of women's satisfaction with maternity care', *Birth* 16(3): 109–13.

Thune-Larsen, K. B. and Moller-Pendersen, K. (1988) 'Childbirth experience and postpartum emotional disturbance', *Journal of Reproductive and Infant Psychology* 6(4): 229–40.

Welburn, V. (1980) *Postnatal Depression*, Glasgow: Fontana.

Wilkes, A. (1990) 'Post-baby blues that lead to breakdown', *The Independent*, 31 July.

Chapter 5

With women
New steps in research in midwifery

Mary J. Renfrew and Rona McCandlish

Research in midwifery has been developing steadily over the past twenty years, during which midwives have been responsible for a wide range of studies. Many of these have investigated areas of clinical practice which midwives believe are important to child-bearing women, such as perineal care (Sleep 1990), labour ward practices (Garforth and Garcia 1987) and postnatal care (Murphy-Black 1989).

In this chapter we describe our experience of running a study which gave us the opportunity to do research *with* women as participants, rather than *on* women, as subjects. Two aspects were especially different and challenging. First, the research question was raised jointly by women who are members of a user group representing childbearing women (the National Childbirth Trust), and by midwives; so there was a shared research agenda. Second, the study was organized with midwives in clinical practice and National Childbirth Trust (NCT) members as active collaborators.

The study, a multi-centre randomized controlled trial, was set up to investigate the effectiveness and safety of treatments for women with inverted and flat (non-protractile) nipples who want to breastfeed; 7–10 per cent of women have inverted or flat nipples on one or both sides (Hytten and Baird 1958; Alexander 1991). Recruitment was organized through two networks, one run by midwives in clinical practice and the other by volunteers in the NCT. In the process of running this trial several issues have been raised about sharing the responsibility for conducting research with midwives in clinical practice and members of a user group. Some of these issues are discussed in this chapter.

Background to the study

Breastfeeding is not always easy. It has been clear for some years that although many women want to breastfeed, they encounter both physical and emotional difficulties and have to give it up before they wish to (Martin 1978; Martin and Monk 1982; Houston 1983; Solberg 1983; Martin and White 1988). Some of these problems arise from help and advice which we know to be inappropriate (Inch and Renfrew 1989), others because we do not yet know the best way to deal with the difficulties experienced by women. A government-sponsored initiative to increase the numbers of women who continue to breastfeed successfully was started in 1988 (Department of Health 1988), and a number of recent publications (Royal College of Midwives 1988; Renfrew *et al.* 1990; Royal College of Midwives 1990) are aimed to improve the information available. However, further research is still needed to address the continuing difficulties which women experience with breastfeeding.

One of the problems which remains to be solved is how best to help women with inverted and flat (non-protractile) nipples. For breastfeeding to be done effectively and without nipple pain and damage, the baby needs to draw the nipple to the back of his or her mouth while feeding (Gunther 1945; Woolridge 1986). Thus breastfeeding is especially difficult if the mother has inverted or flat nipples because these can become sore; and soreness is the commonest reason for stopping breastfeeding in the early days after birth (Martin and White 1988). Two treatments for inverted and flat nipples have been in common use in this and other countries for some years. Neither of these has yet been tested properly. Breast shells were first developed by Harold Waller, an obstetrician, in 1946. These are glass or plastic domes which fit over the nipple inside the bra and if worn during pregnancy are supposed to draw out the inverted or flat nipple. Hoffman's exercises were also developed by an obstetrician, in 1953 and require the pregnant woman gently to stretch the tissue at the base of her nipple several times a day, with the intention of improving protractility.

There is marked disagreement among those who work with pregnant women in the UK and other countries about the value of the two treatments described above. Some insist that their preferred method is essential, others are equally certain that the treatments are damaging to the success of breastfeeding. Although this debate has been going on for many years (for example Ministry of Health 1944), there is, as yet, no clear evidence on which to base advice to women who want to breastfeed.

Origins of the study

In 1985 Jo Alexander, a midwife teacher from Southampton, started to plan a randomized controlled trial to test the effectiveness of breast shells and Hoffman's exercises. She wanted to find the best way to help women with inverted or flat nipples because she herself did not know what treatment to recommend.

Randomized controlled trials

Randomized controlled trials (RCTs) are considered to be the best way to distinguish real differences between the effects of alternative forms of care. Without random allocation to treatments, bias cannot be ruled out as an explanation for apparent differences. Large enough numbers are needed in each group to prevent one being misled by chance differences (Meinert 1986; Chalmers 1989). Although it was traditionally seen as a research method which lay firmly in the domain of medical research, awareness is growing of the need to use this method to answer questions of safety and effectiveness both in terms of 'hard' outcomes such as mortality and physical morbidity, and 'soft' outcomes such as women's views of different forms of care (Richards and Chalmers 1987; Oakley 1990). It is a valuable method in the evaluation of midwifery practice, where both types of outcome are important.

Extending the trial

Alexander and her colleagues started their trial in 1986, but after one year of recruitment it was clear that although the Southampton midwives were recruiting good numbers of women, it would take many years for that one centre to reach the sample size judged necessary to answer the question with confidence. Alexander approached the National Perinatal Epidemiology Unit (NPEU) for help in extending the trial to other centres. The NPEU is a Department of Health funded research unit with extensive experience in organizing trials of clinical practice, including midwifery trials.

There were a number of factors in the decision to extend this trial through the newly-funded Midwifery Research Initiative in the NPEU, where we work. One of the objectives of the Midwifery Research Initiative was to evaluate specific midwifery practices, and we wanted to carry out a randomized trial which examined a common practice. We also wanted to build on the good work already done by the midwives in Southampton. The planned study examined a condition which could be diagnosed and treated by women themselves, and the principal outcome, duration of breastfeeding, could be reported by women fairly easily.

We were approached around the same time by representatives of the NCT, who also wanted to help in answering this question. The NCT is a user group with approximately 40,000 members, which runs antenatal classes and provides breastfeeding counselling and postnatal support services (Kitzinger 1990). Some of its members and staff were concerned about the conflicting information given to women with flat and inverted nipples. They too needed to know what treatment, if any, for inverted and flat nipples was worth recommending. Midwives and members of a user group thus had a shared research agenda. Finally, the proposed trial offered an opportunity for those involved in screening and recruitment, and in being recruited, to be active, acknowledged collaborators. Research could be carried out with women, rather than on women.

Organization of the trial

Planning for the multi-centre trial started in late 1988, and was funded by the Department of Health in early 1989. The study is known as the MAIN trial, an acronym derived from the full title, 'The Multi-centre Randomized Controlled Trial of Alternative Treatments for Inverted and Non-protractile (flat) Nipples in Pregnancy'. Based on Alexander's original protocol, the trial is designed to test the differences between four different groups: breast shells, Hoffman's exercises, a combination of shells and exercises, and a control group who use no treatment to prepare their nipples in pregnancy.

The MAIN trial is organized in two parts. In one, recruitment is organized by midwives in nine centres throughout England. In the other, recruitment is organized through the network of the NCT. Trial organization on both sides is co-ordinated by the Midwifery Research Initiative at the NPEU in Oxford.

There were two reasons for this approach. First, it was calculated on the basis of information available at the time the trial was designed that to demonstrate an 80 per cent chance of a true difference of 10 per cent in the success of breastfeeding at six weeks after birth, a sample size of at least 600 was required. The 'power' of 80 per cent would be increased to 90 per cent if the sample size could be doubled. This would mean screening a minimum of 40,000 women, to find enough women who fulfilled the entry criteria and who might be willing to participate in the trial. Thus we needed an extensive screening exercise; using both the health service and the NCT network increased the number of women who could be screened. Second, we had an interest in the organizational issues involved in carrying out large-scale research with both midwives and women as users of the services. Here we had the opportunity to examine a shared research question which both groups wished to answer. We wanted to build on this interest and goodwill to explore the practical issues in running a research study together with these two groups.

The core planning group at the NPEU designed the trial, and prepared the written material in consultation with midwives, child-bearing women and NCT members and staff. Recruitment was designed to involve the midwives and NCT volunteers as much as possible.

Organizing the midwife-coordinated trial

After initial publicity, we were approached by midwives from nine hospitals in England who wished to participate in the study. In each hospital, a volunteer midwife co-ordinator was identified, to take responsibility for the trial at local level. A network was established in each centre, involving midwifery managers, antenatal and community midwives, to organize effective screening, and recruitment and randomization of women who were eligible to join the trial. Each midwife co-ordinator also identified certain midwifery colleagues as deputies or designates, some to take responsibility for the trial in certain areas, others to stand in when she was not available. All initial training and publicity was carried out jointly by the NPEU midwives and the local co-ordinators. Before the trial started in each centre we tried to talk with as many midwives in antenatal and community care as possible, both formally and informally. We explained the trial, described the procedures and documentation, and responded to any questions or problems. It took a total of six months to start screening and recruitment in eight of the nine centres. The ninth centre, which approached us for information later than the others, began recruitment some months later.

During the preparation, we stressed that the midwives themselves were responsible for the trial, and that their involvement would be fully acknowledged. Each centre developed its own systems of communication and organization, based on the common protocol. Variations in local circumstances, communication and management structures, and social circumstances of the women attending for antenatal care were all taken into account. At the time of writing, the centres have been involved in the trial for a range of three to twelve months.

Women are screened by midwives on a one-to-one basis during the course of routine antenatal care. Women who wish to breastfeed and who fulfil the other pre-established entry criteria (for example, between 26 and 35 weeks of pregnancy, expecting one baby, not having breastfed previously for more than seven days), are asked to examine their nipples, together with the midwife. If their nipples are inverted, this can be seen on inspection. If not, they are asked to carry out a 'pinch test' to check for flat nipples. Checking for flat and inverted nipples in this way is often a part of routine antenatal care.

If a women is eligible, and agrees to enter the trial after discussion with the midwife, the local midwife co-ordinator is contacted by telephone by the recruiting midwife. The co-ordinator randomizes the women to one of the four trial groups by opening a sealed, opaque randomization envelope prepared for the trial by the NPEU. The recruiting midwife then tells the woman about her allocation, gives her any information she may need, and breast shells if that was her allocation.

Organizing the NCT-coordinated trial

Planning for the NCT trial was carried out in collaboration with NCT headquarters staff and officers. Eighteen volunteer local co-ordinators offered to participate, all of them planning to take on this role in addition to NCT involvement as breastfeeding counsellors. One of these volunteers agreed to be the national co-ordinator for the volunteers.

The existing national network of the NCT includes its national magazine *New Generation*, local branch news-letters, antenatal classes, information from breastfeeding counsellors and from the NCT booking clerks who communicate with women booking for antenatal classes. This network has been used to communicate information about the trial. Women learn through this network that if they wish to breastfeed, and have inverted or flat nipples (shown by carrying out the 'pinch test') they can telephone their nearest local co-ordinator for further information. The co-ordinator checks the eligibility criteria in discussion with the woman, then randomizes her to a trial group by opening a sealed, opaque randomization envelope prepared for this trial by the NPEU. The co-ordinator then sends information and breast shells as needed to the women participating. Recruitment on the NCT side of the trial has been running for about twelve months.

Follow-up of all women

Follow-up on both sides of the trial is carried out by the NPEU. Trial entry forms are sent to us by the co-ordinators immediately after recruitment, and we send out a postal questionnaire to women at six to eight weeks after the expected date of delivery. A variety of systems have been set up locally to ensure that women who experience a stillbirth or infant death are not sent questionnaires. The questionnaire booklet contains questions about the duration of full and partial breastfeeding, problems with breastfeeding, women's feelings about the use or non-use of trial treatments, whether or not they carried out their treatment allocation, and what they felt about the trial in general. As well as the more structured questions, there is plenty of space in the questionnaire booklet for women to write about their own experiences, in their own words.

Involving women: information and consent

On both sides of the trial, women who are interested in participating are given information about the trial and what will be expected of them, before they agree to take part. Written information is given to back up a discussion with either an NCT co-ordinator, or a midwife. It is made clear that it is not known which is the best course of action to take for inverted and flat nipples, so there is genuine doubt about whether the treatments being tested are helpful, are harmful or make no difference either way. It is explained that in the light of the present lack of evidence, we really do not know whether it is better for women to receive allocation to an active treatment, or to the control group. In these circumstances, the most ethical approach is to offer treatment in the context of a randomized trial (Chalmers 1986), and this is discussed with all women who are interested in the trial.

Women who do not wish to participate in the trial, or who express a preference for one or other allocation group, are not pressured in any way to take part.

Recruitment to the MAIN trial

At the time of writing, only a third of the expected numbers of women have been recruited to the midwife-coordinated trial. On the NCT side, recruitment has been even slower. As a result, we have examined the problems we have encountered in organizing research in this way.

Challenges in organizing the MAIN trial

Any randomized trial, especially when it involves many centres, has inherent problems. The resulting data can only be relied on with confidence if randomization is carried out properly, and if sufficient numbers of participants are recruited into the trial. In the case of a multi-centre trial, researchers can seldom be on the spot to solve problems, ensure consistency and encourage motivation. This trial has proved especially challenging in giving responsibility for the local organization to midwives in clinical practice, who often have little or no time to spare because of pressures of work, and to NCT members, who are voluntary, have young children and often have paid jobs as well. Neither group has previous experience of being so responsible for running randomized controlled trials. At the time of writing, we have just begun formal evaluation of the research processes involved in this study. The discussion below is a preliminary look at some of the issues we are facing.

Communication

Ensuring accurate, timely and effective communication through both the NCT network and the health service network is a big challenge. Some examples of the methods of communication we have used include specially prepared posters for clinics and antenatal classrooms; information sheets for pregnant women and for midwives using attractive cartoons to convey the central message; gestational calculators with information about the trial printed on the back; a press release to professional and women's journals and magazines; regular telephone contact from the NPEU to all co-ordinators; regular visits by the NPEU staff; meetings of the co-ordinators as needed; and pocket-sized summaries of the protocol which can be carried around by anyone involved in screening and recruitment.

The midwife-coordinated trial depends on midwives who work in the antenatal clinics and in community care to screen and recruit women. At any one time, about 550 midwives work in these areas in the nine participating hospital and community centres. However, many more midwives than this have been involved in the trial over time, as the routine rotation, or changing, of midwives from place to place throughout the hospital and community is now common.

In the NCT-coordinated trial, the nature of the organization inevitably makes communication slow. The NCT has 350 local branches, approximately 40,000 members, runs classes for 15,000 pregnant women each year, has 600 breastfeeding counsellors and 600 antenatal teachers, plus many other volunteers working in a variety of posts. The trial depends on information moving through this network to the local level. Local NCT branches have no hierarchical structure, and rely on the voluntary commitment and goodwill of large numbers of women with young children.

Not carrying out breast examinations

A crucial part of the protocol involves identifying women with flat or inverted nipples. Inverted nipples can be seen on inspection, but the woman needs to test herself for non-protractile, or flat nipples. Alexander's work suggests that of the 7–10 per cent of women with flat or inverted nipples, 20 per cent have inverted nipples, while 80 per cent have flat nipples. If the test for flat nipples is omitted, then up to 80 per cent of potentially eligible women will be unaware that they may be able to participate in the trial.

In the midwife-coordinated trial, the protocol asks midwives to ask the women to examine their breasts, and to carry out the 'pinch test' if necessary. However routine examination of women's breasts is not always offered as part of routine antenatal midwifery care. It is not clear when this practice declined (see for example Hitchman 1971), but midwives we have talked to attribute its discontinuation to a number of recent factors: information available recently about the lack of evidence supporting the benefit of antenatal treatments (for example Royal College of Midwives 1988); lack of time in antenatal visits; and in some places the decreased involvement of midwives in the provision of clinical antenatal care. As a result, a number of the midwife centres in this trial had to introduce antenatal breast examination as part of the research protocol. Some found this easier to implement consistently than others, and we have had to encourage midwives in some hospital and community clinics to ask women to carry out the test.

In the NCT-coordinated trial, the test for inverted and flat nipples is widely publicized through the NCT network. Women are asked to carry out the test themselves, at home. We have encountered difficulties related to communication, and to conveying negative messages, as we describe below. If women do not know about the test, they cannot carry it out, and they will not be able to participate in the trial.

Conveying positive messages about breastfeeding

Some midwives and NCT counsellors and teachers describe a reluctance to give pregnant women any negative messages about their potential ability to breastfeed. Women should start to breastfeed, they argue, with confidence in their own bodies. They are therefore reluctant to discuss the trial with women in case they transmit doubt about the woman's ability to breastfeed successfully. This difficult issue raises questions about how to advise women who may in fact have increased difficulty because of inverted and flat nipples. How do we evaluate the best treatments for them if we cannot discuss the trial?

How important is breastfeeding?

Although there has been increasing attention given to breastfeeding in recent years, and although it is known to be an important issue for women (Laryea 1980; Houston 1983), ambivalent attitudes to breastfeeding are noticeable.

In the midwife-coordinated trial, we have noted that those concerned with antenatal care do not always view breastfeeding as important. We have observed this in antenatal midwifery care, and in the attitude of obstetricians to the trial. Often other priorities and the lack of time at antenatal visits result in little if any discussion of breastfeeding.

In the NCT-coordinated trial, this issue is much less noticeable on the part of the organizers: it is clear that the NCT is committed to breastfeeding, although traces of the same problem have emerged at times. For example, at first the trial was seen primarily as the responsibility of the Breastfeeding Promotion Group (BPG), rather than an important challenge for the whole organization, and as a potential benefit for all women. News about it was given in the BPG news section of *New Generation* and local news-letters. For those without a special interest in breastfeeding, it was possible to miss the publicity altogether. This has now changed, and it is becoming clearer that the organization as a whole has to be involved in the trial to make it a success.

On both sides of the trial, women who might be potential participants seem to be affected by embarrassment and ambivalent attitudes. Recruitment has been adversely affected by the problem that women may not want to discuss whether or not they have inverted or flat nipples. We have encountered both midwives and NCT counsellors who are hesitant to ask women to test their nipples, and this has inevitably slowed down recruitment. Many pregnant women, and some midwives, report a reluctance even to discuss the trial because of the feelings that it engenders. This inhibition in discussing inverted nipples has been described to us as stronger than the reluctance to discuss, for example, perineal care.

Ambivalent attitudes to breastfeeding among women themselves and those who work with childbearing women are widespread (McIntosh 1985; Renfrew 1988), and not new. We are just recovering from the havoc wreaked by writers from the past, many medically qualified and male, who advocated regimens for breastfeeding which were totally inappropriate (Pritchard 1904; Vincent 1904; Truby King 1924). Some women writers, however, did not help much. Midwifery writers tended to follow medical advice (Liddiard 1923; Myles 1975; Bailey 1976). Often not mentioned at all by early feminist writers, breastfeeding was seen by some as another tie to women's traditional roles (Firestone 1980; de Beauvoir 1983). Artificial feeding was seen as part of women's emancipation (Reiger 1988), and at least one feminist text on mothering (Chodorow 1978) ignores breastfeeding as an issue for women at all.

Recent writers have challenged these views, noting that women often experience deep feelings of distress in wanting to breastfeed but encountering difficulties (Laryea 1980; Filshie *et al.* 1981; Houston 1983). Some writers have described breastfeeding as a powerful attribute and a special part of women's sexuality (Newton 1973; Kitzinger 1979; Palmer 1988; Reiger 1988).

In spite of this, breasts are still endowed with the rather sleazy image associated with pornographic magazines, leaving many women reluctant to breastfeed even in normal social circumstances (McIntosh 1985; Joint Breastfeeding Initiative 1990). It is not surprising therefore that women and those caring for them find inverted and flat nipples a difficult topic to discuss, or that this has had an impact on the MAIN trial recruitment.

Feelings about randomized controlled trials

Feelings about randomized trials among midwives and NCT members are mixed. Some accept the usefulness of the method, and the need to allocate randomly when information is not known about the effectiveness and safety of treatments. Others believe in the benefits of one or other treatment being tested, or conversely believe that the treatments cause harm, in spite of the lack of evidence. It becomes very hard for people with strong feelings either way to encourage randomization, or to randomize. This trial depends on the involvement of large numbers of midwives and NCT members and inevitably some of them hold strong feelings one way or the other. As a result some of those involved in the recruitment process may be reluctant to discuss the trial, and women who might be interested in participating may not even be told about it. This feeling is not, of course, confined to midwives and NCT members. Members of the medical profession, social scientists and members of the public have expressed similar feelings (Faulder 1985; Chalmers and Silverman 1987; Oakley 1990; Korn and Baumrind 1991).

Feelings about research in midwifery

Midwifery research is relatively new. The Midwifery Research Database (MIRIAD 1990) has records of 129 studies. Only one of these studies was started before 1975, twenty-two between 1975 and 1980, with gradually increasing annual numbers up to 1990. There are reports of a few early studies not yet entered on this database (for example Ministry of Health 1949; Auld 1974), but these are rare. It seems fair to conclude that interest and activity in the field of midwifery research really started in the 1970s and gained momentum in the 1980s.

Consequently, the development of a culture which encourages midwives to read, use and conduct research is relatively recent. Midwives are not used to asking their own questions and taking responsibility for answering them. This has raised a number of problems for us in organizing this trial.

For example, the trial started around the time of clinical regrading, when morale among the midwifery profession, and the relationship with managers, was severely strained (*Nursing Times* 1988a, 1988b, 1988c). Midwives asked us how we could consider midwifery research to be important, when the real battle concerned the midwife's role.

We have also found that midwives providing antenatal care often cannot find the time to spend on the screening and recruitment necessary for the MAIN trial. This may be related to tiredness and overwork (see below), but it is also because of the priority given to the other tasks they are doing. These may include more clerical tasks than clinical work, and we have found that many midwives are not able, or expected, to spend time with individual women in antenatal clinics.

In spite of the fact that most midwives have extensive experience of gathering data for someone else's research, very few have so far been involved in carrying out research for which they have primary responsibility. They often collect data for other research studies, either national or local. These are usually medical research studies, and midwives report that they have seldom been asked in advance if they are willing to act as routine data collectors. A clash of values has been described to us over the importance attached to medical research as opposed to midwifery research. We have encountered both midwives and doctors who argue that priority should be given to medical research, as well as midwives who are committed to this trial, and who believe that they should take responsibility for their own midwifery research.

We have talked with some obstetricians and also with some midwives in clinical practice and in management who are not convinced that midwives can, or should, do their own research. Indeed, there is little incentive for midwives to take on the extra work needed to do this. For example, the criteria used to determine the clinical grading for midwives do mention *participation* in research, stating that in some senior posts (H and I grades only) the midwife may be expected to 'participate(s) in research, and/or equipment testing' (Nursing and Midwifery Staffs Negotiating Council 1988). *Initiation* of research is only mentioned in the criteria for a Clinical

Specialist. There is no indication that midwives at grades below H (senior midwife sisters are often graded G) are expected to participate in research at all.

Some doctors and midwives, we have found, attach little importance to the research questions which midwives ask. Though this may, in part, be related to a lack of familiarity with research in midwifery, there seem to be other issues. These relate to the power structures both within midwifery and between midwifery and obstetrics, similar to those described by other authors (Robinson *et al*. 1983; Robinson 1990).

Midwifery management support

One of the most important factors influencing the midwife-coordinated trial has been the amount and type of support from midwifery management. Without this support, centres cannot sustain recruitment. In some centres, the local co-ordinator has been released from some of her normal responsibilities, while in others she has been expected to carry out the trial on top of an already difficult work-load. Some managers take a personal interest in the trial and see it as a challenge for all the midwives in the hospital and community. Others see it as a drain on already scarce resources, and are frankly sceptical or indifferent. Again, this issue seems to be related to the value placed on midwifery and midwifery research.

Lack of time, and tiredness

It is clear that the midwives with whom we have had contact carry extremely heavy work-loads. There is virtually no spare capacity within the system to build in extra research time. Midwifery research is simply not part of the work that midwives are expected, or expect, to do. This issue is closely linked with the value placed on midwifery research as described above, as it is apparent that gathering information for other research studies is something that midwives are expected to find time to do and accept as part of their work-load.

Women working as volunteers within the NCT have only limited energy to spare for projects such as this. This energy can only be tapped fully at certain times of year, and Christmas and school holidays have a noticeable adverse effect.

Future strategies

We have designed a number of new strategies, based on some of the information discussed here, which we have learned in the course of running the trial. Recruitment seems to be increasing as a consequence. We are also conducting a formal survey of the issues in organizing research in this way, where midwives and user group members take responsibility for running a trial.

As a result of our experience with this trial so far, we have several difficult questions to ask ourselves about organizing research with midwives and with service users as active collaborators.

1 Can midwives in clinical practice, and volunteer mothers, organize a large trial? Or does overwork and lack of time inevitably get in the way?
2 Is research done by midwives, and by childbearing women, inherently less valuable than that done by doctors? If not, why does it seem to be viewed as such?
3 How can we best communicate difficult and emotional issues and information about a trial around two very large and diffuse networks?
4 How can we address the markedly ambivalent views of breast-feeding in this culture?

We hope to address some of these questions in the remaining months of the trial.

Acknowledgements

We would like to acknowledge the time, commitment and input of all midwives and NCT members involved, and of the women recruited on both sides of this trial. Barbara Henry, Jane Moody and Mary Newburn of the NCT made collaboration with their organization possible. We are grateful for helpful discussions with Iain Chalmers, ongoing assistance from Adrian Grant and Diana Elbourne, and the support and advice of all others in the NPEU. Jo Alexander carried out the original work on which this trial is based, and has supported the development of this trial. Sheena James and Ursula Bowler have contributed to its successful administration. The trial is funded by the Department of Health, England.

References

Alexander, J. (1991) 'The prevalence and management of inverted and non-protractile nipples in antenatal women who intend to breastfeed', submitted PhD thesis, University of Southampton, Human Reproduction and Obstetrics, Faculty of Medicine.

Auld, M. (1974) *How Many Nurses?*, London: Royal College of Nursing.

Bailey, R. (1976) *Mayes Midwifery*, 9th edn, London: Balliere Tindall.

Chalmers, I. (1986) 'Minimizing harm and maximizing benefit during innovation in health care: Controlled or uncontrolled experimentation?', *Birth* 13: 155–64.

Chalmers, I. (1989) 'Evaluating the effects of care during childbirth', in I. Chalmers, M. Enkin, M.J.N.C. Keirse (eds) *Effective Care in Pregnancy and Childbirth*, Oxford: Oxford University Press, 3–38.

Chalmers, I. and Silverman, W. A. (1987) 'Professional and public double standards on clinical experimentation', *Controlled Clinical Trials* 8: 388–91.

Chodorow, N. (1978) *The Reproduction of Mothering: Psychoanalysis and the Sociology of Gender*, London: University of California Press.

de Beauvoir, S. (1983) *The Second Sex*, Penguin Modern Classics edn, Harmondsworth: Penguin.

Department of Health (1988) *Caring for the Breastfeeding Mother: 'The Lost 25 Per Cent'*, London: Department of Health.

Faulder, C. (1985) *Whose Body is it? The Troubling Issue of Informed Consent*, London: Virago.

Filshie, S., Williams, J., Osbourn, M., Senior, O. E., Symonds, E. M., Baskett, E. N. M. (1981) 'Post-natal care in hospital – time for a change', *International Journal of Nursing Studies* 18: 89–95.

Firestone, S. (1980) *The Dialectic of Sex*, London: The Women's Press.

Garforth, S. and Garcia, J. (1987) 'Admitting – a weakness or a strength? Routine admission of a woman in labour', *Midwifery* 3: 10–24.

Gunther, M. (1945) 'Sore nipples – cause and prevention', *The Lancet* 2: 590–3.

Hitchman, M. (1971) 'Breast feeding' (letter) *Midwives' Chronicle and Nursing Notes*, January: 24.

Hoffman, J. B. (1953) 'A suggested treatment for inverted nipples', *American Journal of Obstetrics and Gynaecology* 66: 346–8.

Houston M. J. (1983) 'Home support for the breastfeeding mother', in: M. J. Houston (ed.) *Maternal and Infant Health Care, Recent Advances in Nursing*, Edinburgh: Churchill Livingstone, 49–69.

Hytten, F. E., and Baird, D. (1958) 'The development of the nipple in pregnancy', *The Lancet* 2: 1175–7.

Inch, S., Renfrew, M. J. (1989) 'Common breastfeeding problems', in I. Chalmers, M. Enkin, M. J. N. C. Keirse (eds) *Effective Care in Pregnancy and Childbirth*, Oxford: Oxford University Press, 1375–89.

Joint Breastfeeding Initiative (1990) *Breastfeeding Survey*, London: National Childbirth Trust.

Kitzinger, J. (1990) 'Strategies of the early childbirth movement: A case-study of the National Childbirth Trust', in J. Garcia, R. Kilpatrick, M.

Richards (eds), *The Politics of Maternity Care: Services for Women in Twentieth-Century Britain*, Oxford: Clarendon Press, 92–115.

Kitzinger, S. (1979) *The Experience of Breastfeeding*, Harmondsworth: Penguin.

Korn, E. L. and Baumrind, S. (1991) 'Randomised clinical trials with clinician-preferred treatment', *The Lancet* 337: 149–52.

Laryea, M. (1980) 'The midwife's role in the care of primigravidae and their infants during the first 28 days following childbirth', M. Phil. thesis, Newcastle Polytechnic.

Liddiard, M. (1923) (reprinted in 12 edns until 1948) *The Mothercraft Manual*, London: J. & A. Churchill.

Martin, J. (1978) *Infant Feeding 1975: Attitudes and Practice in England and Wales*, London: HMSO.

Martin, J. and Monk, J. (1982) *Infant Feeding 1980*, London: HMSO.

Martin, J. and White, A. (1988) *Infant Feeding 1985*, London: HMSO.

McIntosh, J. (1985) 'Barriers to breastfeeding: Choice of feeding method in a sample of working class primiparae', *Midwifery* 1: 213–24.

Meinert, C. L. (1986) *Clinical Trials: Design, Conduct and Analysis*, Oxford: Oxford University Press.

Ministry of Health (1944) *The Breastfeeding of Infants*, Report of the Advisory Committee of Mothers and Children, Public Health Medical Subjects Report 91, London: HMSO.

Ministry of Health, Department of Health for Scotland, Ministry of Labour and National Service (1949) *Report of the Working Party on Midwives*, London: HMSO.

MIRIAD (1990) *Midwifery Research Database, First Annual Report*, Oxford: National Perinatal Epidemiology Unit.

Murphy-Black, T. (1989) 'Postnatal care at home: A descriptive study of mother's needs and the maternity services', unpublished paper, Nursing Research Unit, Department of Nursing Studies, University of Edinburgh.

Myles, M. (1975) *Textbook for Midwives*, 8th edn, Edinburgh: Churchill Livingstone.

Newton, M. (1973) 'Interrelationships between sexual responsiveness, birth and breastfeeding', in J. Rubin and J. Money (eds) *Contemporary Sexual Behavior*, New York: Johns Hopkins University Press.

Nursing and Midwifery Staffs Negotiating Council Handbook (1988) Amendment to Section 2, Clinical grading review: grading definitions, issued under advanced letter (NM) 1/88.

Nursing Times (1988a) News item, 84(43): 3 and 9.

Nursing Times (1988b) News item, 84(48): 5.

Nursing Times (1988c) News item, 84(49): 5.

Oakley, A. (1990) 'Who's afraid of the randomized controlled trial? Some dilemmas of the scientific method and "good" research practice', in H. Roberts (ed.) *Women's Health Counts*, London: Routledge, 167–94.

Palmer, G. (1988) *The Politics of Breastfeeding*, London: Pandora Press.

Pritchard, E. (1904) *The Physiological Feeding of Infants*, London: Henry Kimpton.

Reiger, K. (1988) 'Women's bodies, women's rights', *Breastfeeding Review* 13: 29–30.

Renfrew, M. J. (1988) 'What we don't know about breastfeeding',

Breastfeeding Review, 13: 105–10.

Renfrew, M. J. Fisher, C., Arms, S. (1990) *Bestfeeding: Getting Breastfeeding Right For You*, Berkeley, Calif.: Celestial Arts.

Richards, M. and Chalmers, I. (1987) 'Intervention and causal inference in obstetric practice – how have things changed over the past ten years?', *New Generation*, March: 6–8.

Robinson, S., Golden, J., Bradley, S. (1983) *A Study of the Role and Responsibilities of the Midwife*, Nursing Education Research Unit Report No. 1, London: London University.

Robinson, S. (1990) 'Maintaining the independence of the midwifery profession: A continuing struggle', in J. Garcia, R. Kilpatrick, M. Richards (eds) *The Politics of Maternity Care: Services for Childbearing Women in Twentieth-Century Britain*, Oxford: Oxford University Press, 61–91.

Royal College of Midwives (1988) *Successful Breastfeeding*, London: Royal College of Midwives.

Royal College of Midwives (1990) *Helping a Mother to Breastfeed: No Finer Investment*, video, London: Royal College of Midwives.

Solberg, S. M. (1983) 'Indicators of successful breastfeeding', in M. J. Houston (ed.) *Maternal and Infant Health Care: Recent Advances in Nursing*, Edinburgh: Churchill Livingstone, 26–48.

Sleep, J. (1990) 'Perineal care: a series of five randomized controlled trials', in S. Robinson and A. M. Thomson (eds) *Midwives, Research and Childbirth*, Vol. 2, London: Chapman and Hall, 199–251.

Truby King, F. (1924) *The Expectant Mother and Baby's First Months*, London: Macmillan & Co.

Vincent, R. (1904) *Nutrition of the Infant*, London: Balliere Tindall & Cox.

Waller, H. (1946) 'The early failure of breastfeeding', *Archives of Disease in Childhood* 21: 1–12.

Woolridge, M. W. (1986) 'The anatomy of infant sucking', *Midwifery* 2: 172–6.

Chapter 6

'My health is all right, but I'm just tired all the time'
Women's experience of ill health

Jennie Popay

In general men experience higher death rates than women in every age group from birth through to old age, whilst women consistently record higher levels of illness than men. (For recent reviews see Verbrugge and Wingard 1987; Whitehead 1987.)

This general picture is, however, complicated when one looks at different types of ill health, or morbidity as it is technically termed, and different age groups. In the middle years of life, for instance, gender differences in recorded chronic illness are significantly reduced. Males have higher rates of serious illness whilst the excess ill health amongst females appears to be largely in relation to non-life-threatening physical conditions, various measures of mental illness and poor subjective perceptions of health status in general. Women also have higher consultancy rates, particularly in relation to general practice. However, if account is taken of consultations for pregnancy, childbirth and diseases of the genito-urinary systems, the female excess virtually disappears (Macfarlane 1990). The intricacies of these patterns and in particular the female excess on what some see to be less 'valid' measures of illness has lead to the argument that women's experience of minor illness is not 'real'.

Women are most likely to report more ill health than men on two types of measures: subjective measures, in which people are asked whether they have experienced a particular symptom, for example, and measures of restricted activity, in which people are asked if they have had to limit the things they do because of an illness. To simplify somewhat, it is argued that women will be more likely than men to respond positively to these types of questions because they are more sensitive to their own and other people's experience of illness and because the social roles they occupy – notably those of full-time housewife or mother – give them more freedom to limit their activities when they are 'feeling ill'. (See for example Nathanson 1975; Verbrugge 1976; Verbrugge 1977; Mechanic 1978; Verbrugge and Wingard 1987.) According to this argument therefore, women's higher rates are not a measure of an excess of 'real' illness compared to men, but rather are created by the research design.

In this chapter these types of explanations for sex differences in the experience of health and illness are critically examined from a sociological perspective. It will be suggested that such explanations are too simplistic because they fail to take account of the meanings men and women attach to the experience of ill health, and what these can tell us about the subjective reality of their daily lives. Using qualitative data I seek to illustrate how accounts of the experience of tiredness can enrich our understanding of the processes which may generate gendered differences in the experience of health and illness.

The study

The data presented in this chapter were collected during a larger study of patterns of health and health care behaviour amongst women and men with dependent children. The study involved two related dimensions: secondary analysis of existing large data sets and in-depth case-studies of a year in the life of women and men in eighteen households in the London area. The data presented here are drawn mainly from the household case-studies, but the tables draw on data from the Health and Life-styles Survey 1984–5 (as described in Cox et al. 1987) and the OPCS General Household Survey.

Case-study research is by its nature small-scale and intensive. The focus is not on discovering how many and what kind of people in the general population have particular characteristics. Rather it explores the meanings people attach to their experiences and identifies and describes the social structures and processes that shape these meanings.

A particular focus of the case-study research described in this chapter was to consider whether there are aspects of the experience of parenthood which all women and men share and others which divide them. We were therefore concerned with the cross-cutting axes of gender, class and race. The case-study households were chosen to facilitate this objective. In particular the material circumstances of the households varied considerably, from those living on supplementary benefit to those living on incomes in excess of £100,000 a year. In this way we were able to consider how and to what extent material living standards enable women and men to reduce the burden of parenthood and other roles, and what if any were the limits to this. The number and ages of children varied from one to three and from a baby born during the study to young people aged 18 years. Fifteen of the households included two parents and in three of them there were mothers alone. Two households included black women and men. Finally there was variation in the employment status of both women and men.

The case-study households were obtained through three different channels: from a larger survey of households in London, from a London general practice register and through personal contacts, though none of the households was known to the researcher at the beginning of the study. The aim was to have at least three interviews with each household member over the year. However, in three of the eighteen households only one round of interviews was obtained and in another household the mother withdrew after the first interview. Complete data are therefore available on fourteen households. The interviews were always conducted separately with men and women and all covered a range of issues, including the respondents' experience of health and illness in the past and during the period of the study. The interviews were largely unstructured, with the respondent raising many of the issues within the general context of their experience of being parents. Tiredness as an issue was raised in a variety of contexts but most commonly, as we shall see, in relation to accounts of parenthood in general or to how the respondents felt their health had been in the recent past.

The problem with explanations for sex differences in the experience of ill health

A dominant explanation for the female excess of minor illness compared to men is that this excess is not real but simply a reflection of women's greater propensity to report and act on symptoms. These arguments relate to two different dimensions of the experience of ill health: an individual's experience of symptoms and his or her behaviour in response to these.

Much existing research on sex differences in the experience of ill health, and the explanations that have grown out of this work, are underpinned by the assumption that there are objectively identifiable categories of illness or symptoms to be experienced and acted upon which are in some sense more real than people's subjective accounts of them. From this perspective, the excess of ill health reported by women is argued to be the result of the way ill health is measured in research. The female excess in ill health is most apparent on measures which rely on self-reports of symptoms and which focus on behaviour in response to illness. It is therefore argued that because women are more sensitive to illness and pain and are more likely to report and act upon symptoms than men, they will inevitably have higher rates on these types of measures, but these are not measures of 'real' illness.

The literature on gender inequalities in ill health is full of examples of this type of reasoning, much of which was reviewed and criticized in 1979 by Gove and Hughes (1979). This paper was itself subsequently criticized by Marcus and Seeman (1981) on the grounds that it relied on self-report measures of illness rather than measures of 'real' illness. Most recently Verbrugge, who has published widely in this field, and Wingard similarly concluded that,

> A strictly medical view of the data leads to a simplistic conclusion that 'females are sicker than males and they have greater disability, health service use and drug use because of that'. But when we acknowledge social factors we see that higher female morbidity rates may result from their illness prevention orientations and health reporting behaviour, not necessarily from greater real morbidity. Because males have higher inherited and acquired risks of illness, it is likely that real morbidity rates are actually higher for them for many diseases. And for diseases with real female excess, social factors act to boost the sex differences.
>
> (Verbrugge and Wingard 1987: 135)

The social factors referred to here are the differences in reporting behaviour and responses to symptoms discussed above.

These arguments raise two intriguing questions. First, is it the case that women are consistently more likely than men to report and act on symptoms? Second, is it sociologically acceptable to reject findings based on subjective measures of ill health as less 'real' than findings based on more objective measures, and therefore of no theoretical interest?

Research findings bearing on the question of whether women are more likely than men to report and act on symptoms are patchy and inconclusive. In their 1979 literature review for example, Gove and Hughes argue that there is an impressive array of evidence to suggest that women are no more likely to do so than men and that the existing literature presenting the arguments 'is based on the beliefs of the authors who provide the appearance of empirical support for their assertion by a process of mutual citation' (Gove and Hughes 1979: 128). In their review of this literature, Verbrugge and Wingard also acknowledge that whilst there is a widespread belief that men and women differ in what these authors term their 'illness and prevention orientation' the evidence is limited (1987).

Research has suggested that women in different social roles – the unmarried compared to the married, for example, those with children compared to those without, and those with paid employment compared to full-time housewives – behave differently in relation to illness. However the relationship is complex and may vary depending on the outcome measure used (see, for example, Nathanson 1975; Jenkins 1985; Rosenfeld 1989). More important however, because much of this research includes only women, it casts little light on possible differences in the illness orientation of men and women, and it contributes little to our understanding of gendered patterns of morbidity and illness. It is possible that men's willingness to report and act on symptoms will similarly vary according to the number and nature of the social roles they occupy. But women may still experience more ill health overall.

The arguments that women's social roles provide them with more opportunity to respond to illness than do men's have tended to focus on the lack of time constraints on women's lives. However, it is clearly the case that women who combine the roles of housewife, mother and paid employee have less free time than either employed men or full-time housewives. It would also appear to be the case that full-time housewives work longer hours per week on average than employed men (Kowarzik and Popay 1988). Verbrugge and Wingard argue that the crucial feature may be the flexibility in women's social roles rather than the amount of free time:

> More flexibility in time schedules does not necessarily mean that women have more leisure time than men . . . it can simply mean they can be more flexible in whatever schedule they have; they can take time off from a job or housework more easily.
>
> (1987: 132)

As they note, however, such an assertion remains to be demonstrated. In relation to our first question then, it is apparent that more research is needed on differences in men, and women's willingness to report and act on symptoms and on the difference, if any, in the degree of flexibility experienced by men and women in different social roles.

What then of the second question: Is it appropriate to reject findings of a female excess of self-reported or behaviourally linked measures of ill-health as of no theoretical interest to debates about gender inequalities in ill health? Sociological research has shown that definitions of what constitutes illness, disease or health vary according to a range of social, cultural, economic and historical factors. As Clarke has argued,

> It may be that rates of illness are different for men and women not because men and women have a different proclivity for this 'objective' phenomenon, but rather because illness means something quite different to the members of each sex.
>
> (1983: 71)

From a sociological perspective these different categories of meanings should become the focus of research concerned to identify and understand the social processes which generate the differences. It follows from this that research on gender inequalities in health and illness should not be primarily concerned with whether the patterns of ill health amongst men and women reflect 'real' or 'true' differences. Rather it should be exploring whether particular symptoms or experiences do mean something different to men and women. Neither is it enough to stop at the point of identifying different categories of meaning. Research should also be concerned to explore what these differences tell us about the nature of social relationships.

There is a growing volume of work on the meaning of illness, though little of this deals directly with categories of meanings amongst men and women. According to this research it would appear that the process of defining oneself as ill or deciding to act on the symptoms depends in part on how common a symptom is in a society or group. If a symptom is common, it is more likely to be considered normal and therefore not defined as illness. In his study of illness behaviour, for example, Zola (1966) found that tiredness was often considered normal and therefore not defined as illness. Similarly, Fox (1968) found that while backache was considered abnormal amongst people in higher socio-economic groups and was therefore likely to be viewed as illness, amongst people in lower socio-economic groups it was considered to be an inevitable part of life.

A second important factor in the process of defining oneself as ill is the extent to which a symptom 'fits' with the major values of a society or group. The definition of illness, it is argued, is culturally constructed. Zola (1966), for example, suggests that differences in the illness behaviour of Irish and Italian immigrants to America were due to cultural differences. Whilst Italians' behaviour was marked by expressiveness and expansiveness, the Irish tended to ignore and underplay bodily complaints.

Cultural patterns may, however, vary depending on the social context in which symptoms occur. The expectations of the people experiencing the symptoms, in terms of how others will respond to their being ill, are important, as too are the costs and benefits associated with defining oneself as ill. Blaxter's (1982) work on definitions of health amongst working-class women in Aberdeen illustrates the importance of the social context of symptoms. For these women to 'be healthy' meant to be able to function in one's social roles as housewife, mother and so on. Regardless of the presence of symptoms, if one is able to continue paid and unpaid work then one is not ill. Cornwell's work on lay accounts of the causes and consequences of ill health also points to the dominant influence of the social context on beliefs about health and illness (Cornwell 1984).

Research therefore suggests that the process of defining oneself as ill and deciding what action if any to take – that is, the meanings people attach to particular symptoms or signs – are in an important sense socially constructed. In making visible the factors which shape these meanings, research is also making visible the social relationships, structures and roles in which individuals are embedded and which determine to a greater or lesser extent their experience of health and illness.

What then is the experience of tiredness among women and men, and what if anything can this tell us about the links between gender relationships and roles and the experience of ill-health amongst women and men? First the relative rates of tiredness reported in large survey research are considered, followed by accounts of tiredness and of behaviour in response to symptoms provided by a small group of women and men. These accounts are explored in order to identify in what ways the meanings attached to tiredness and illness behaviour vary by gender, material living standards and other social factors, and to ask what this can tell us about the processes underlying the female excess of minor illness.

Tiredness and gender differences in the meaning of illness

As one commentator has recently noted, 'fatigue is the normal chaff of living' (Ridsdale 1989: 486). In a now somewhat dated diary-based study, for example, women aged between 20 and 40 recorded 400 episodes of tiredness for every one brought to a physician (Banks *et al.* 1975). Tiredness is undoubtedly a complex, multi-faceted phenomenon. In some instances it may be a mild, transitory experience, in others a severe and chronic one. It may be a sign of psychological disturbance or the presence of a physiological disorder (Wessely *et al.* 1990). The cause may be readily identifiable from a medical perspective, or impossible to isolate. Tiredness therefore epitomizes many of the problems inherent in the study of the meanings of symptoms. The frequency with which it is reported and the sex differences in the patterns found in large-scale surveys also mean than a study of tiredness may tell us a great deal about sex differences in the experience of ill health.

In a recent national survey in the United Kingdom involving a sample of some 9,000 women and men aged over 18 around 20 per cent of men and 30 per cent of women reported 'always feeling tired' in the month before the interview (Cox *et al.* 1987). Similarly in a Danish survey involving a sample of over 1,000 40-year-olds, 41 per cent of the women and 25 per cent of the men reported feeling 'tired at the moment' (Norrelund and Holnagel 1979). Tiredness

Table 6.1 Proportion of women and men aged 18–39 reporting 'always feeling tired', by presence, age and number of children

	Women		Men	
	%	number	%	number
No children in household	31.3	233	19.8	162
Age of youngest child:				
under 1 yr	39.4	122	20.0	42
1–5 yrs	38.2	236	22.7	85
6–16 yrs	31.1	266	19.6	87
Numbers of children:				
1 child	32.2	119	20.0	43
2 children	34.1	217	21.7	83
3 or more children	35.9	107	21.9	33

Data from Health and Life-styles Survey 1984–5 [Cox *et al.* 1987]

therefore, like many other minor symptoms, shows a female excess. Beneath these gross figures, however, the experience of tiredness also varies in interesting ways amongst women. As Table 6.1 shows, amongst women aged under 39, those without children and those with children aged 6–16 are less likely to report 'always feeling tired' than those with younger children. Similarly as the number of children increases, so does the proportion of women reporting tiredness. Though a similar pattern is evident amongst men the differences in the rates are minuscule: the presence, age and number of children has little if any impact on the level of tiredness reported by men. So what meanings do women and men attach to these experiences?

Accounts of tiredness amongst women and men

Amongst the eighteen women and fourteen men in the case-study households, tiredness was one of the most frequent symptoms or conditions spontaneously referred to. Most respondents commented on their experience of tiredness at some point during the interviews, but the women were more likely to do so than the men. More important, however, there appeared to be two very different types of accounts of tiredness which, though not confined exclusively to men or women, were gendered.

The first type of account was provided by all but two of the men who talked about tiredness and by five women. In these accounts tiredness was presented as a minor or intermittent event which was a normal part of life and basically not a cause for concern. Amongst the men in particular, it was often linked to paid work, either in terms of the hours or the pressure of work.

> Over the last 4–5 years the hours have got longer . . . I don't particularly mind the week . . . I do find at the weekends I sleep quite a lot . . . It's quite tiring, especially if you go out in the evening. I mean you find yourself awake from 6.30 till . . . I mean we got to bed last night at one o'clock . . . some people can do it, I can't. So I get quite tired.
>
> (Father)

In contrast, the second type of account was provided by most women and two men, one in a dual-career household, taking relatively equal responsibility for the care of two young children, the other a man in his early sixties (considerably older than any of the other respondents). Here, tiredness was described as a severe or chronic experience. These accounts, illustrated by a single quote below, were provided by women with very different household situations in terms of the number and age of children, their employment status and their standard of living:

> The worst thing is the tiredness, the exhaustion ... by the end of the day ... you're too physically exhausted to do anything.
> (Part-time employed mother, two parents, 3 children: 6 months, 3 years and 6 years, high income)

Only in a few instances had this severe tiredness triggered a visit to the doctor and for this to happen it would appear that tiredness had to be combined with other symptoms. In these circumstances it became a sign that there might be something more serious wrong. These cases occurred in both women and men. The 'participative' father in the dual-career family, for example, had reported during the first interview that he was tired all the time. During the third interview he described how he had been to the doctor because,

> I felt fairly tired and light headed actually. I thought I was going to faint at one stage ... they did some blood tests and I've still got to have some more because one showed that there might be something not standard with the liver.

These few instances apart, and despite the severity or persistence, the second type of tiredness, like the first, was also presented as a 'normal' feature of everyday life:

> I think you probably don't let yourself think about it ... because it's no good going around saying 'Oh I feel tired' ... it's probably just a natural hazard of the world we live in.
> (Full-time housewife and mother in two-parent household with two children aged 5 and 7, and full-time nanny)

Though considered to be normal, this severe or chronic tiredness was clearly seen to be a consequence of the way their lives were organized. The man in the dual career household, for example, explained that he had 'no time to relax'. Similarly, the mother of three children in a middle-income household who also had a part-time evening job said,

When I had Daniel I wasn't tired because I had nobody else to run around, but when I had Daniel and then I had Tracey, then there was a difference, I was tired and then I went in for Sarah and I had two to run after, then I *was* tired. But I also get tired if they wake me up in the night or I'm up early or I work one night.

Different types of tiredness amongst women

Women were more likely then men to report severe tiredness but accounts of severe tiredness were not confined to any particular type of household. There were, however, some subtle variations in the accounts of severe tiredness provided by women living in different circumstances, which are worthy of note. The notion of different types of tiredness has been reported from other qualitative research. Brannen and Moss (1988), for example, have argued that women's experience of tiredness varies in type as well as quantity, according to different stresses in different situations. Young babies and broken nights brought one type of tiredness; being at home full time was likely to induce another, centred on lethargy and boredom; trying to combine domestic and paid work was linked to a third type, derived from physical and mental fatigue.

There are some similarities, but also differences, in the types of tiredness described by the women in the case-study households compared to Brannen and Moss's study. This is perhaps not surprising given that the case-study group are much more diverse in terms of the age and number of children and their social and economic circumstances. Both of the lone mothers, for example, linked their tiredness to the physical demands of lone parenthood, but also to their psychological state. This link was not evident in any of the other severe tiredness accounts. Liz was a lone parent of 23 with one 3-year-old child. When talking about her experience of being a mother she felt that she lacked patience and consistency because of tiredness. This in turn she linked to lone parenthood: 'I think it's 'cos I'm on my own now, it is that bit harder. It does get me down more than before.'

At a later interview, however, she made the following statement: 'I think tiredness can be linked to depression . . . like now even though I've got more nights [work] at the pub and I've got my sister's child to look after as well . . . it's like an incentive . . . I feel I've got a lot more life in me now.'

Similarly, Ann, an older lone parent with two teenage children, when asked how she had been since the last interview, replied 'shattered'. She noted that her job was pressured, that she didn't get a break during the day and then rushed home at night 'getting the shopping, the cooking, then cleaning up'. Later, however, she explained that she wasn't sleeping very well because 'my mind does too much overtime, I think that's basically why I'm tired . . . I've got a lot on my mind'.

Though women with older children did report severe tiredness, some of the most vivid and extreme accounts of physical and mental exhaustion were provided by women who had young children now or in relation to the period when their children were small. Here two prominent themes, in addition to broken nights, appeared to be the constant demands made on one's time and energy by small children and the responsibility one has for their welfare and development:

Thomas couldn't go to bed unless he was breastfed and I was exhausted and didn't feel like doing it and it just seemed like all on me . . . he was big enough really to go to bed on his own, but it was just like a habit and . . . he was still acting like a baby . . . you're always alert . . . not completely relaxed . . . Even when they're sleeping . . . because you feel it is your responsibility.

This situation was linked by women not simply to the degree of tiredness, but to its chronicity. Ann for instance gave the following account of the years when her teenage sons were young: 'So we went through the most incredible years of exhaustion . . . he was strong and healthy and we were practically wrecked.'

Similarly, Lorraine with a young baby and two other children under 7 described how in the seven months since the birth she had 'just kept going and knowing in the back of my mind I'd have days when I didn't know if I could get on, you know, put one foot in front of the other. But I mean, I think everyone does that.'

Lorraine was also combining care of three young children with a part-time job, which she acknowledged was an important factor in her physical exhaustion, but which at the same time provided her with mental stimulation: 'I need a lot of stimulation now and getting out helps a lot . . . I think that sitting idle I feel quite boring or bored.' Her reference to the possibility of 'sitting idle' is ambiguous given the pressure she described above and to some extent reflects a devaluing of domestic labour. At another time for example, she described how when she didn't have a paid job she would be constantly cleaning the house.

It was also evident from some women's accounts that physical exhaustion was seen to be part of the price that was to be paid for combining paid work with domestic labour. Linda, for example, had a senior full-time administrative post, as did her partner. They had two children under 6 and a day-time nanny. She noted that she did feel tired a lot of the time, but went on, 'It's mind over matter really . . . you have to learn to cope with it don't you . . . I mean sometimes we think we can't go on like this and we do.'

Another part of the 'price' to be paid for having employment appeared to be a commitment to spending time with the children at a level of intensity not apparent in the accounts of full-time housewives and mothers. Linda carried on to point out that she and her partner hadn't gone out and left the children with a babysitter since their 5-year-old son was born: 'When we're here we're quite child-centred I think . . . at the weekend and the evenings . . . in that we put them first and I suspect they get as much of my time as they might get from other parents.'

Lorraine had a similar commitment:

> I try and keep the time from 3.30 onwards for the children. I don't really clean or do anything like that . . . I mean it's still the quality of the time that you spend with children, not the quantity . . . I'm with them consistently until 7 . . . and I dance and I play with them and I actually do things with them rather than being in another room.

As with the women in Brannen's study, full-time housework and child care were linked in some women's accounts to a different type of tiredness. Ann, for instance, though sharing child care with her husband had no organized or paid activities outside the home on a regular basis at the time of the first interview. She described how, since having children, she could function on less sleep than previously without feeling physically so tired. However, she noted that she now experienced more 'lethargy'. Similarly, other women reported being bored or frustrated with full-time domestic labour and child care.

Severe or chronic tiredness was also reported by women across the social classes. Even women in the most economically advantaged positions reported extreme or chronic fatigue and linked this experience to the demands of their daily lives, albeit at times somewhat ambivalently. Rebecca, for instance, had two children aged 4 and 7. She had a live-in nanny and other domestic help:

I think we are all tired is the answer quite a bit of the time and we all lead terribly hectic lives, even me who is . . . I mean I'm not working or anything but it is all go and we get up and you know quite early and I'm frightfully bad about going to bed . . . I am now going to bed terribly late.

Similarly, Jane, who had two teen-age daughters, a large number of animals to care for and daily domestic help, described periods of intense fatigue when her 'blood [felt] like water'. Asked about the causes she suggested that her daily life contributed to them:

I've been under quite a lot of stress what with one thing and another . . . it's like problems with the children or with Tom's work . . . it's just actually what causes stress is the amount one tries to fit into a day . . . it is literally just pressure trying to push through all that we've got to get through plus other things that crop up in between.

Partners' perceptions: through the looking glass

When men and women talked about their partners' experience of tiredness, the nature and causes of these experiences were not always perceived in the same way. Five of the women whose husbands had given an account of mild tiredness described their husbands' tiredness as severe. In one household, for example, the man reported that he was 'a bit tired sometimes' when he got home from work, whilst his wife reported that, 'He comes home tired, fed up, with headaches and you name it . . . stomach aches, very tired, headaches every day.'

None of the women suggested that her partner's tiredness was less severe than the husband described it and they shared the man's perception that the experience was linked to employment. 'I think he does get very tired, terribly tired, and I'm not surprised . . . and I wonder you know how I can help him but that's his job' (Full-time housewife and mother, with children of 15 and 17, high income).

In contrast some of the men's accounts of their partner's tiredness reflected a degree of scepticism at the possibility that this was a result of the demands of domestic roles.

She's always tired. Well she reckons she needs about 28 hours sleep a day . . . No, she does like sleep. Oh I think the kids are wearing, you know, really all day . . . but I say to her that she's got a cushy life because she can spend the afternoon with friends.

(Father, skilled work with 3 children, aged 2, 4 and 7)

There was only one instance where a husband described a wife's experience of tiredness as more severe than the woman did herself. Though provided as an explanation for why the couple did not often go out together in the evenings, the account is a disarmingly vivid description of the way he perceives his wife's life to be organized:

When you think although Bev is supposed to be in a part-time job, in fact she's probably not getting out sometimes till quarter past three and by the time she's taken the daughter to gymnastics most days . . . and see weekends and that it's housework so she's dead tired of an evening.

It is clear from these data that women in these case-study households were describing a qualitatively different experience from men when they talked about tiredness. Though there were two men who shared this experience, it is interesting that one was more involved in the day-to-day care of his children than most of the other men and the other was much older than the group as a whole. It would also appear that men's experience of tiredness was given more legitimacy by their partners than was the case with women's experience.

Despite the severity of the experiences described, there was no indication that women were more likely than men to define themselves as ill or to take any action to ameliorate the 'symptoms'. Indeed there is evidence from the case-studies that at a more general level women are more reluctant than men to define themselves as ill.

Adopting the sick role: to be or not to be ill

As we have already noted, it has been argued elsewhere that women will report more ill health than men because the social roles they traditionally occupy provide them with a better opportunity to act on symptoms and adopt the sick role. Verbrugge and Wingard (1987) have suggested that the crucial feature of women's social roles may be flexibility. However, far from being an obvious feature, flexibility seems to be missing from the daily experience of life as mother, housewife or paid employee amongst the women in the case-study households.

Regardless of the age of children, the household type, whether or not they had a paid job or their household income, women emphasized that if they felt unwell they would 'pretend it wasn't there', 'just carry on' or keep themselves 'constantly under check'. Some women suggested that they were trying to stop doing this and take better care of themselves, because their illness 'made it very difficult for the family'.

> I just could not move and I had to get somebody in to organise the children and the animals and everything. So constantly after that my husband said 'Don't ever let that happen again'. I mean it's very difficult for them. . . . I think I'm learning, to know myself . . . I stop sooner rather than trying to carry on.

This woman's husband shared her concern, noting that 'When Nicky in particular is ill, there's a big problem.'

Alternatively some women were attempting to change because they felt their behaviour was adversely affecting their health. In one instance, for example, a mother described how she ended up in hospital with pneumonia because she had ignored symptoms for three weeks. However, as the quote below illustrates, women may not find it easy 'taking better care of themselves'.

> When we finished dinner I didn't kind of stretch myself to clean up everything. I went to bed and rested for an hour. I asked him to get me a drink one night . . . I mean I put the children to bed and I didn't ask him to cook dinner and things like that, I could manage that. . . . I have actually realised that I can't push myself all the time.

Like tiredness, the perceived lack of freedom or 'time to be ill' was intimately linked by women to the demands of their various roles. A central feature of these demands was the sense of responsibility they felt towards their children, or their employers, as Lorraine illustrates:

> Unless I'm really ill I still go to work. I would never stay in bed unless like, I mean, I was being sick . . . that's the only reason . . . you know, things get delayed and I still have to do certain things . . . I still have to look after the children . . . lying in bed I just find I worry and I tend to think 'Oh my goodness, what was that noise, I'd better deal with it'. The men are fine, they're just lucky that they can switch off, and it's probably a better thing . . . we're all – women – like that.

As another woman's account illustrates, the intensity of the demands of daily life may divert attention from the experience of the symptoms:

I've found since having children in about six years I think I've only
been in bed maybe twice . . . if I do get a fluey thing I notice it gets
bad in the evening and at night and I tend to sort of sweat it out.
In the daytime I function normally. Whether I just feel that I can't
get them to the extent I had them before . . . I will deal with them
by getting them badly in the evening, but in the daytime, as far as
looking after the kids is concerned, I just carry on.

(Mother, high income, 2 children)

Husbands appeared to agree that women were reluctant to adopt the
sick role. However, there were different perceptions as to why this
might be the case. One idea was that women were in some ways
more stoical or had a greater capacity to cope with pain and stress
than men. As one man put it, 'Women tend to be more resilient, in my
experience they cope with an awful lot of stress and actual physical,
not feeling unwell, you know, monthly period things; perhaps they're
used to coping with it.'

Another explanation was that women behave irresponsibly. One
husband complained that his wife 'won't allow herself to be ill' and
said, 'It's a common trait amongst women, not all but some women,
I think. The more tired they get, the more they try to do.'

Finally, there were those households where there was a perception
that the demands of their daily lives either in the home or at paid work
simply meant that neither of the parents had any time to be ill.

In discussing their own behaviour when they were feeling unwell,
men described a similar reluctance to that described by women when
it came to taking time off from paid employment. However, there
was a tendency for both women and men to agree that once at
home men showed a willingness – indeed at times an eagerness
– to adopt the sick role. Whilst a husband noted, for example,
that 'I will be flat out in bed, demanding everything to be
done for me ... I think generally when men are sick they
think the world has come to an end', his wife commented,
'He's a big baby, he comes home and goes straight to bed.'

Discussion

These data do not, therefore, support the idea that women perceive
themselves as having freedom to be ill, neither is this view shared by
their husbands. Nor do the data support the view that in relation to
the experience of tiredness at least, women are more likely than men

to define themselves as ill. What they do suggest is that the subjective experience of severe or chronic fatigue is linked by women to their experience as housewives and mothers either alone or in combination with other roles. These experiences also appear to have elements in common across social classes.

So what is to be made of these data? The question as traditionally framed would be, 'Are women really more tired than men or are they simply more willing to talk about their tiredness or more sensitive to the physical and phychological concomitants of tiredness than men?' But from a sociological perspective this is not the appropriate question. Even if there were some 'objective' phenomenon called 'tiredness' which could be measured and the scores compared within and across the sexes, would this be more 'valid' or 'accurate' than subjective accounts?

In part, it depends on what the measure is to be used for. Subjective accounts may be more relevant to predicting subsequent behaviour than objective measures. There is also growing evidence that subjective measures of health and illness may be powerful predictors of future mortality and morbidity even in the absence of clinical or physiological risk factors. (See for example Kaplan and Kotler 1985.) But subjective accounts of tiredness can do much more than that. They can also increase our understanding of the nature and causes of differences in men's and women's experience of health and illness.

The meanings attached to the experience of tiredness amongst women and men may, for instance, help us to understand some of the sex differences in ill health reported in large-scale surveys. In the annual General Household Survey, for example, rates of ill health reported by women and men in couple households vary, depending on the measure of ill health being considered, as the data in Table 6.2 illustrate.

Men in couples are marginally more likely to report a long-standing illness whilst women in couples are marginally more likely to report a recent illness. However, the gender gap is widest with regard

Table 6.2 Health status of men and women in couple households

	Men, %	Women, %
Long-standing illness	26	23
Recent illness	9	11
Good health in year	75	68

Source: Popay and Jones 1990, Table 1

to subjective perceptions of good health in general in the past year. Here, it is shown that women are less likely than men to feel their health has been good, despite the marginally lower rate of long-standing illness they report. Some commentators would presumably argue that these data do not reflect 'real' differences in the experience of ill health. However, it could equally be argued that a major factor in explaining why almost a third of married women feel that in general their health has not been good in the past year is the severe or chronic tiredness they experience. It has been argued in this chapter that women are reluctant to define tiredness as an illness, despite its severe character, which means it would not be reported as long-standing or recent illness in response to the GHS question. However, it may well be reflected in women's perceptions of health status in general. As the woman quoted in the title of this chapter succinctly put it, 'My health's all right, but I'm just tired all the time.'

Subjective accounts of tiredness may also tell us something about the way in which gender and health and illness are constructed. At a superficial level these women and men are describing what they believe to be the causes of tiredness, and its significance. However, at another level of analysis they could be seen to be articulating the nature of social – in this case – gender relationships. These accounts reveal not only how women and men think about particular symptoms, but also how they understand the organization of their lives and the social expectations of their roles.

It was suggested earlier, for example, that women were unlikely to define tiredness – no matter how extreme or chronic – as an illness or to assume the sick role in response to this. Several factors may be working to influence this situation, but two are particularly worthy of consideration. First, there are the social expectations attaching to women's domestic labour. Graham (1982) has elaborated the concept of coping as a key component of the role of housewife and mother. To be a successful mother and wife, one must cope; to complain is not to cope and therefore to fail in a social position central to many women's identity and self-esteem. If chronic or severe tiredness is a persistent feature of fulfilling the mother and wife role then it is to be expected that women will feel under pressure to cope with this too, and not to complain.

This analysis also makes sense of the commonality of the experience of severe or chronic tiredness across social classes. Whilst the demands of the mother and wife role and the social and economic circumstances in which she is expected to fulfil them may vary across social classes, the expectation that a woman will cope – with four children under 6 in a damp house, living on income support, or with four dinner parties a week for ten important guests – spans this divide.

A second factor which should be considered when seeking to understand women's accounts of tiredness, is the response of others, notably their partners. Men's own accounts suggest that they were not generally sympathetic to women's experience. To the extent that the adoption of the sick role requires the approval of important others, women appear to be less likely to obtain approval from their partners than vice versa. This perspective throws a somewhat different light on Lorraine's comment, quoted earlier, that men are lucky because they can 'switch off' whilst women can't. A somewhat different interpretation of this situation is that men are 'allowed' to 'switch off' by others in the household, whereas women are not.

Essentially, then, what has been argued here is that rather than engaging in a debate about the 'validity' or otherwise of subjective accounts of ill health and health, sociologists should be paying more attention to the theoretical potential inherent in these accounts. As Joan Scott has argued, 'Language is not simply words in literal usage, but the creation and communication, in particular context of meanings – through allusion, metaphor and especially through differentiation' (Scott 1987: 15). It is, in the final analysis, an old argument: a call to listen and take seriously what people say.

Acknowledgements

The research on which this paper was based was undertaken as part of the ESRC-funded programme of research within the Centre for Studies in Education and Family Health, an ESRC-designated research centre in the Thomas Coram Research Unit (TCRU). I am grateful to the parents who have taken part in the research and to the OPCS and the ESRC Data Archive for the use of the General Household Survey and the Health and Life-styles Survey. Thanks are also due to Gill Jones for comments on the draft, Olwen Davies the project secretary, to Charlie Owen, Senior Programmer at TCRU for his advice and assistance with software for qualitative analysis, to Sandra Stone who typed the chapter, and to Gill Bendelow, a student on the project, who helped in the data collection.

The data in Table 6.1 are taken from work on the Health and

Life-styles Survey presently being undertaken by the author as part of an ESRC-funded study of work roles and women's and men's health, Grant no.: R000 23 1774.

References

Banks, M., Beresford, S., Morrell, D. (1975) 'Factors influencing demand for primary medical care in women aged 20–44 years: A preliminary report', *International Journal of Epidemiology* 4: 189–95.

Blaxter, M. (1982) *Mothers and Daughters: A Three Generational Study of Health Attitudes and Behaviour*, London: Heinemann.

Brannen, J. and Moss, P. (1988) *New Mothers at Work: Employment and Child Care*, London: Unwin Hyman.

Clarke, J. (1983) 'Sexism, feminism and medicalism: A decade review of literature on gender and illness', *Sociology of Health and Illness* 5(1): 62–82.

Cornwell, J. (1984) *Hard-Earned Lives: Accounts of Health and Illness from East London*, London: Tavistock.

Cox, B., Blaxter, M., Buckle, A., Fenner, N., Golding, J., Gore, M., Huppert, R., Nickson, J., Roth, R., Stark, J., Wadsworth, M., Whichelow, M. (1987) *The Health and Life-styles Survey: A Preliminary Report*, Cambridge: Health Promotion Research Trust.

Fox, R. (1968) 'Illness', in K. Sills (ed.) *International Encyclopaedia of the Social Sciences*, New York: Free Press.

Gove, W. and Hughes, M. (1979) 'Possible causes of the apparent sex differences in physical health: An empirical investigation', *American Sociological Review* 44(2): 126–46.

Graham, H. (1982) 'Coping or how mothers are seen and not heard', in S. Friedmarsh and E. Sarah (eds) *On the Problems of Men*, London: The Women's Press.

Helman, C. (1984) *Culture, Health and Illness*, London: John Wright & Sons Ltd.

Jenkins R. (1985) 'Sex differences in minor psychiatric morbidity', *Psychological Medicine* monograph, supplement no. 2.

Kaplan, C. A. and Kotler, R. L. (1985) 'Self-reports: Predictive of mortality', *Journal of Chronic Diseases* 38: 195–201.

Kowarzik, U. and Popay, J. (1988) *That's Women's Work*, London: London Research Centre.

Lewis, G. (1981) 'Cultural influences on illness behaviour', in L. Eisenberg and A. Kleinman (eds) *The Relevance of Social Science for Medicine*, Dordrecht: Reidel, 151–62.

Macfarlane, A. (1990) 'Official statistics and women's health and illness,' in H. Roberts (ed.) *Women's Health Counts*, London: Routledge, 18–62.

Marcus, A. and Seeman, T. (1981) 'Sex differences in health status: A re-examination of the nurturant role hypothesis' (Comment on Gove and Hughes ASR February 1979) *American Sociology Review* 46: 119–23.

Mechanic, D. (1978) 'Sex, illness, illness behaviour and the use of health service', *Social Science and Medicine* 9: 57–62.

Nathanson C. (1975) 'Illness and the feminine role: A theoretical review', *Social Science and Medicine* 9: 57–62.

Norrelund, N. and Holnagel, H. (1979) 'Fatigue amongst 40 year olds', *Ugeste Laeg*: 1425–9, quoted by H.G. Kennedy, 'Fatigue and Fatigability', in *The Lancet* (1987) 1: 1145.

Oakley, A. (1974) *Housework*, Harmondsworth: Penguin.

Popay, J. and Jones, G. (1990) 'Patterns of health and illness amongst lone parents', *Journal of Social Policy* 19(4): 499–534.

Ridsdale, L. (1989) 'Chronic fatigue in family practice', *Journal of Family Practice* 29(5): 486–8.

Rosenfeld, S. (1989) 'The effects of women's employment, personal control and sex differences in mental health', *Journal of Health and Social Behaviour* 30: 77, 91.

Scott, J. W. (1987) 'On language, gender and working class history', *International Labour and Working Class History* 31 (Spring): 1–13, University of Illinois.

Verbrugge, L. (1977) 'Females and illness: Recent trends in sex differences in the United States', *Journal of Health and Social Behaviour* 17: 387–403.

Verbrugge, L. (1977) 'Sex differences in morbidity and mortality in the United States', *Social Biology* 23: 275–96.

Verbrugge, L. (1985) 'Gender and health: An update on hypotheses and evidence', *Journal of Health and Social Behaviour*, 26: 156–82.

Verbrugge, L. and Wingard, M. (1987) 'Sex differentials in health and mortality', *Women and Health* 12(2): 103–43.

Wessely, S., Nickson, J., Cox, B. (1990) 'Symptoms of low blood pressure: A population study', *British Medical Journal* 301: 362–5.

Whitehead, M. (1987) *The Health Divide*, London: Health Education Council.

Zola, I. (1966) 'Culture and symptoms: An analysis of patients presenting complaints', *American Sociological Review* 31: 615–30.

Chapter 7

'Isn't she coping well?'
Providing for mothers of triplets, quadruplets and quintuplets

Frances Price

To conceive, deliver, nurture and care for triplets, quadruplets, quintuplets or more is an extraordinary situation for any woman to confront. Despite an increase in recent years, such higher-order multiple births remain uncommon and unexpected.

Faced with three, four or more infants of the same pregnancy, what is to be expected? Tina Perridge's imagery featured in a newsletter for other 'supertwin' parents, when her triplets were 2 years old:

> Having survived the endless feeds, chaotic nights and the ultimate lunacy of taking triplets out on reins, I have come to the conclusion that life as a parent of triplets takes on a certain unique quality – rather like riding a bicycle, juggling eggs and whistling a song all at once!
>
> (Perridge 1985)

Another mother of triplets, Kathy Topping, who had initiated the newsletters, had earlier called attention to the difficulties of securing suitable help. She wrote, 'I do feel that you just cannot cope alone' (Topping 1983).

One hundred and eighty-three sets of triplets, eleven sets of quadruplets and one set of quintuplets were born in England and Wales in 1989, compared with seventy sets of triplets and six sets of quadruplets in 1982: 28.6 sets per 100,000 deliveries in 1989 compared with 12.2 per 100,000 in 1982. As fertility drugs (Schenker *et al*. 1981) and assisted conception techniques, such as *in vitro* fertilization and embryo transfer (IVF) and gamete intrafallopian transfer (GIFT) have contributed to this increase, the rise in numbers can be expected to continue (ILA 1990; MRC 1990).

Also, more triplets and quadruplets now survive than was the case in the 1970s and earlier. But their mortality rates have not fallen as rapidly as those for single births (Botting *et al.* 1987). Complications of prematurity and uteroplacental insufficiency are the main contributors to perinatal morbidity and mortality (Hays and Smeltzer 1986). Infants delivered at a multiple birth are at an increased risk of cerebral palsy, particularly spastic diplegia (Stanley 1984; Patterson *et al.* forthcoming).

This chapter draws from a project intended to elucidate the problems faced by parents who care for triplets, quadruplets and quintuplets. Some of the dilemmas of study design are explored. The substance of the chapter interweaves qualitative data from the study with supplementary data from three other surveys. The focus is the paradox inherent in the idea of mothers 'coping' with triplets, quadruplets and quintuplets.

Few women and men envisage the situation. Nor can they imagine the magnitude of the responsibility, or the consequences and costs of caring for these children. The familiar is rendered unfamiliar and the effects may overwhelm, not only because of the sheer number of infants born, but also because there is no structured provision for the cumulative consequences, once mother and babies are discharged from hospital.

For various reasons, anticipated levels of help may not be elicited from friends and relatives, or be reliably proffered by others. Such is the novelty of the situation and scale of the demands that the help, support and advice available from the health and social services, and also from the voluntary sector, may not begin to meet the needs as perceived by the parents. Moreover these services are already stretched, both as a consequence of welfare policies transferring care to the community and a shortage of volunteers.

The struggle of mothers to cope is compounded by an administrative limbo and professional uncertainty and disunity. Social workers, health visitors and volunteers, variously empowered to assist, may feel disturbed by their inability to provide or summon up the help and support required. Sympathetic contact by professionals or volunteers may cease. Community resources may never be made available. Three of the twenty sets of triplets in Syrop and Varner's study required placement in foster homes (Syrop and Varner 1985).

The Parents' Study, in the National Study of Triplets and Higher Order Births

This chapter draws largely from the findings of the Parents' Study, a national research project involving the mothers, and many of the fathers, of triplets, quadruplets and quintuplets who were born in the United Kingdom in the years 1979–88 (Price 1989). Above all, the study was intended to obtain information about the specific needs and problems of these parents, their sources of assistance, advice and benefits in kind. Parents' own views about the type, quality and timing of the help and support were central to the study. Beyond this, the aim was to suggest how the care and support given to these families by health authorities, local authority social service departments and voluntary agencies might be better targeted.

Funded by the Department of Health, the Parents' Study is one of a series of complementary surveys of obstetricians, medical specialists, general practitioners and parents. Together, these surveys comprise the National Study of Triplets and Higher Order Births (the National Study) (Botting *et al.* 1990). Colleagues at the Office of Population Censuses and Surveys (OPCS) in London, at the Child Care and Development Group (CCDG) at the University of Cambridge and the National Perinatal Epidemiology Unit (NPEU) in Oxford collaborated in the venture.

The idea of a national study of triplets and higher order births, and specifically the problems faced by their mothers and fathers, had arisen during conversations in 1983 between David Baum, Martin Richards, Director of the CCDG, and Alison MacFarlane and others of the NPEU core staff.

At that time David Baum was a neonatal paediatrician in Oxford and had been responsible for the neonatal care and subsequent paediatric follow-up of several sets of triplets, including the triplet nieces of Martin Richards. Both paediatrician and psychologist knew about the stress such children impose on their mothers, as well as on any brothers and sisters. Practical advice for parents of twins is available, derived from a considerable research literature on twin development (Bryan 1984; Showers and McCleery 1984; MacGillivray *et al.* 1988). But there was no similarly helpful published research about higher order multiple birth children. Case reports in the medical literature seldom touch on social issues compounding the medical concerns, particularly after the babies come home from hospital.

By comparison with twins, the very unusualness and geographical scatter of triplets or more has precluded systematic study of the consequences for those concerned with their care. A thorough search of the literature revealed only a handful of even remotely relevant references. The most frequent were to the work in the early 1980s of the developmental psychologist, Esther Goshen-Gottstein, which occurred solitarily in disparate bibliographies. Four sets of twins, six sets of triplets and three sets of quadruplets had been observed by Goshen-Gottstein and her assistant 'intensively in their homes' in Israel on regular visits made when the children were aged between 5 months and 42 months. Her concerns were at variance with those being developed here, one of her conclusions being that 'excessive' parenting may be elicited in parents of twins, triplets and quadruplets (Goshen-Gottstein 1980).

The collection of experiential accounts from the children's parents was made a feature of our National Study from the outset. Triplet, quadruplet and quintuplet mothers' evaluations of and commentaries on the support and care they received before, during and after pregnancy and delivery became crucial to the entire project (Graham 1984).

The National Study was envisaged at the outset as a series of complementary surveys. Information was to be collected by postal questionnaire from obstetricians, paediatricians and other specialists, general practitioners and parents. The idea was that each questionnaire should relate to the same population of triplets and higher order births.

The birth registration system for England and Wales was used to identify higher order births in 1979, the pilot year, and in 1980 and 1982 to 1985. The surveys collecting information from obstetricians, paediatricians and general practitioners were conducted jointly by OPCS and NPEU. The survey of parents and the associated interview study, together called the 'Parents' Study', was undertaken from the CCDG. All the surveys were planned and overseen by a steering group including clinicians, two mothers of triplets, and members of the three centres responsible for undertaking different parts of the research programme.

Throughout the research period the National Study was given a high profile. A press statement, entitled 'The trials and tribulations of triplets' was issued at the start of the study. Then, once the content of the protocol had been agreed by the steering group copies were distributed to relevant committees, Royal Colleges and associations for comment, support and, where necessary, approval.

The research programme was not only complex but also crucially dependent on the co-operation of a wide range of interests. Both the British Medical Association and the Cambridge District Ethics Committee gave approval, and the study was welcomed by professional and voluntary organizations, including the Royal Colleges of Obstetricians and Gynaecologists, of General Practitioners, and of Midwives, the National Childbirth Trust and the Twins and Multiple Births Association (TAMBA). Fired by our own enthusiasm and buoyed up by the welcome that news of the study seemed to elicit, we underestimated the difficulties of obtaining the practical participation of individual clinicians and general practitioners in completing questionnaires about the mothers and their children.

Early in 1985 the pilot work for the Parents' Study began, and I contacted mothers and fathers of triplets and quadruplets through friends, colleagues and press reports. I arranged informal interviews with them and the two mothers of triplets on the steering group in their homes and discussed their experience of having triplets or quads and of the care of three or more children of the same age, often in addition to older children.

In October 1985, following this exploratory work, a research proposal was submitted to the Department of Health and Social Security (DHSS) requesting funding for the Parents' Study. The proposal was costed to come within the Department's Small Grants Scheme, intended for research projects costed at less than £40,000, and was accepted under the scheme in February of the following year. However, because the complementary surveys collecting information from obstetricians and general practitioners were not yet underway, the start of the Parents' Study was postponed until July 1986.

The procedure

Briefly, the research procedure was as follows. Questionnaires were sent to consultant obstetricians about each triplet and higher order birth, and about matched singleton and twin births as control groups. For each multiple birth there was a questionnaire about the mother and a questionnaire about each baby. If three or more of the babies had been discharged from hospital, questionnaires relating to the mother and to each of her triplets, quadruplets or more were sent to her registered Family Practitioner Committee to be sent on to her general practitioner. We could not initiate direct contact with mothers' doctors.

None of us anticipated the complications that would be introduced at this stage. General practitioners reacted variously; some sent the entire package of questionnaires, worded for them to complete as medical professionals, apparently unread, to the mothers themselves, startling them with a request that they complete them; others summoned the mother to the surgery so that together they might complete the questionnaires; some doctors wrote to OPCS demanding payment to complete; others returned the package uncompleted to OPCS with a note to the effect that they were too busy, or that it was 'a busy time of year' (see Wilmott 1987). Formally, a mother could not be consulted about her willingness to be included in the Parents' Study until she was, in fact, already included in the surveys collecting information from obstetricians and general practitioners. The Family Practitioner Committee with whom she was registered was identified using the National Health Service Central Register. Only through this route was it possible to locate her doctor and thence her. But the general practitioner had the power of veto. Contact could only be attempted if, in her doctor's opinion, there was no overriding reason why her address should not be made available to the researchers working on the study.

If the general practitioner did complete the questionnaires as requested and decided to release the mother's address, a copy of the Parents' Study questionnaire could be posted to her, together with a letter of explanation and reply-paid envelope from me. This was the official route of access to each mother to request her participation in the study. She could not be contacted first to ask her consent. The ethical dilemma could not be resolved but the members of the steering group believed that, to an extent, it could be alleviated.

In the attempt to compensate for our inability to contact mothers directly, the steering group promoted widespread publicity about the project. Apart from the press release at the outset, two annual newsletters were circulated. In June 1987 there was widespread publicity in the national press. *The Daily Telegraph*, the *Guardian* and the *Daily Mirror* carried news items and *The Times* and *The Independent* carried features. Mothers and fathers of triplets, quads or more were encouraged to contact OPCS if they wished to take part in the study. This early publicity together with subsequent magazine articles gave rise to a steady flow of enquiries, not only from parents but from local authority managers, directors of community nursing, health visitors, hospital social workers, field social workers and home care organizers. This high profile enhanced the response not only to the Parents' Study but also to the three other surveys from which this chapter draws.

The crucial factor in the progress of this study was the enthusiastic support from mothers of triplets and quadruplets and also many fathers who wrote, or with whom there was telephone contact. Some contacted OPCS directly. Others were contacted via an intermediary or by following up their details from a newspaper feature, to ask if they would like to take part in the study. The publicity we obtained worked powerfully as an additional dynamic in establishing the collaboration between myself and in particular the mothers of triplets and more.

The steady flow of new names and addresses which resulted could, however, surmount only in part the dependence of this study on the progress of the surveys of obstetricians and GPs. Delays in the completion of these surveys significantly delayed the Parents' Study. Belated completion of obstetric questionnaires meant that the flow from obstetrician to GP to parents was interrupted. There was insufficient time within our grant-funded study period to contact most of those parents whose addresses were obtained only in the spring of 1989 as a result of late responses to the GP survey. Meanwhile, the continuing publicity meant that other parents, particularly those whose triplets or quads had only recently been born, or were shortly to deliver, contacted OPCS or CCDG and asked for information about the study.

Interviews and questionnaire response

An important part of the design of the Parents' Study was that the interview programme was tied to the pattern of questionnaire return. We determined a method for the selection of a sample to interview which took account of the time pressures on the Parents' Study and enabled interviewing to start whilst questionnaires were still being sent out and returned. Two regionally differentiated lists of respondents were compiled in order to accommodate well-documented differences between the north and the south of the country in terms of gross weekly earnings, income support, free school meals, consumer durables and also access to infertility services.

Basing our calculation on obtaining at least 250 questionnaire respondents, it was agreed that every fifth respondent on each list would be approached with a request for an interview, and that the counting should begin with a random number. This ensured that the first five respondents on each list had an equal chance of inclusion in the study. In addition fourteen interviews were conducted with those mothers who requested that I complete their questionnaires with them in their homes. In total seventy-two interviews were obtained with the mothers and sometimes also the fathers of triplets, quads and quins born in the years 1979–88.

Surveys of provision by statutory services

In November 1986 the DHSS requested a survey of both the Health and Personal Social Services as to the support they could provide following triplet and higher order births and the problems they perceived.

These two questionnaire surveys were undertaken in the latter part of 1988 with follow-ups in the spring of 1989. The response from the Social Services departments (132 in all) was initially slow: only 57 replies had been received by the second week in December 1988, a response rate of 43 per cent. Reminder letters together with second copies of the questionnaires were sent out in the first week of March 1989. As a result 102 completed questionnaires were obtained by the time of computer entry in mid-May 1989, a response rate of 77 per cent.

To survey health authority provision, all district health authorities in England, Wales and Northern Ireland and all Health Boards in Scotland, a total of 216, were sent a questionnaire between the last week of September and the first week of December 1988. Reminders were send out in March 1989. The number of usable responses received in time for computer entry was 196, a response rate of 91 per cent.

Both surveys revealed substantial variation in the level of service provision and highlighted the practical difficulties of finding resources to meet the specific needs of these households. Additional material was enclosed with the questionnaire which powerfully supported the magnitude of needs described by the parents, particularly from those in the health and personal social services who, collectively or individually, were involved in the welfare of these families.

The impact on health

In response to the question 'Did you or your partner have any problem with your health in [the] first year?', one mother of triplets wrote in her questionnaire 'Not exactly – just felt very tired all the time. Did suffer from some depression in early weeks.' However, in her response to another question she made clear that she did tell her doctor about the state she was in, but refused the anti-depressants offered her, because she believed her depression to be the result of lack of sleep. Other mothers responded that neither they nor their partners had any problems with their health. But some then wrote 'Tired' beside the question.

Whilst the National Study was underway, junior hospital doctors complained vociferously about their sleep deprivation. An editorial in *The Lancet* entitled 'The dangers of not going to bed' reviewed the legal controls and research findings for pilots, lorry drivers and soldiers (*The Lancet* 1989). Soldiers on exercise are impaired by a single night without sleep (Haslam 1982). Sleep-deprived doctors report mood changes, including anger, hostility and sadness (Orton and Gruzelier 1989). Mood changes, the editorial observes, reflect a wider stress syndrome attributed to sleep deprivation.

Tiredness was the most common condition mentioned in relation to health and illness in Jenny Popay's interview study described elsewhere in this collection. In her study, however, tiredness seldom precipitated a visit to the doctor. Only where other symptoms compound the situation, Popay suggests, is tiredness likely to be reported to the doctor.

Reports of sleep deprivation extending well beyond the early months were uppermost in many of the women's accounts. A mother of triplets and one older child described her exhaustion:

I got to the stage when I felt exhausted. I'd wake up in the morning feeling exhausted. Every day I woke up having had a decent – well, a long night's sleep, feeling more and more exhausted. And I started going to bed on Saturday afternoons, and I'd still feel exhausted. And I started to feel very tense in my arms and legs, they sort of ached, and I felt as if I was struggling to put one foot in front of the other, and I felt awful. And people tell me now that I looked awful. But I felt as if I looked awful as well. And I used to spend sort of hours sitting in the kitchen in tears because they'd trodden in the cat's saucer or something like that. The least little thing they did would just spark it off.

Many of those interviewed made it clear that a strong motivation to participate in the study was the desire that others did not go through a similar experience. Some women voiced their fears about, and in a few cases described the consequences of, their own or their partner's lack of control under stress.

Help with feeding and child care at night was seldom provided from statutory sources. A very small proportion of the households which included triplets, and less than half of the quadruplet and quintuplet households, had received health or local authority night nurse provision, or a night sitter, for any period at all.

Only a third of Directors of Nursing Services in the survey of community nursing provision confirmed that there was the possibility of night nurse provision. Several directors remarked that it had been possible only in 'extreme' or 'very special' circumstances, where 'parents have been unable to cope' or where there were 'considerable social problems':

> We have not provided night nurses where triplets have been involved and would not for quads, unless there was a nursing need. The help required in such a household with normally developing infants would be to satisfy a social need. However, we have on one occasion provided nursery nurse support to a family who fell into the category of 'higher order births', where prior to the birth, an elder sibling had been the subject of Case Conferences covered by Social Services under the Child Abuse Procedures. In this instance, help provided by our Department allowed for 5 nights per week up to 40 hours between 10.00 p.m. and 7.00 a.m. for 6 months, and Social Services provided home help input in the day.
> (Questionnaire response, UK Community Nursing Services Survey, November 1988)

One hundred and three mothers (38 per cent of all triplet mothers) reported that they (27 per cent), or their partners (4 per cent), or both of them (7 per cent) had a problem with their health in the first year after the birth of their triplets. Half of the quadruplet mothers reported health problems in the first twelve months; eight wrote of problems with their own health, two noted problems with their partners' health and two described both their own and their partners' health problems.

'Terrible' and 'dreadful' featured in the mothers' and fathers' written accounts. Stress-related disorders, frequent infections, total exhaustion and depressive conditions of varying degrees of severity predominated.

> I suffered from depression after the children's birth and came very near to a nervous breakdown within a month of them coming home.

> Both permanently tired. After 2 years I was treated for depression.

> Exhaustion mainly – lack of sleep. Dreadful backache.

> Permanent fatigue, particularly from night feeds.

> My husband was off work 3 weeks advised by his doctor through lack of sleep. [His] work was suffering. I suffered postnatal depression for 3–4 months.

> I suffered terrible depression about 3 weeks after arriving home, coupled with complete exhaustion.

> Stress! (i.e. skin disorders and migraine). Back problems lifting them all the time.

> Started with rheumatoid arthritis due to exhaustion. Gastric stomach. Depression (related to stress).

The written replies to other questions displayed the extent to which ill health and chronic depression in the first year were under-reported, as were accidental injuries. At least two fathers fell down flights of stairs whilst carrying one or more of their triplets, with resulting injury to all of them which required hospital treatment. The mother who reported 'I suffered from depression and was always tired. My husband broke his arm', was unusual in including information about a bone fracture in her questionnaire.

Only a third (31 per cent) of the respondents to the UK survey of community nursing provision to these households envisaged any special health visitor input, and one mother of triplets, a health visitor herself, spoke of her disquiet about this:

> [Having] talked to other mothers of triplets throughout this country, I am quite horrified at the lack of health visitor input. That they've had to struggle to a clinic. Not had support at home from the health visitor. Not had support from the midwife. Really been left to get on with it.

She emphasized the importance of a follow-up visit after diagnosis as an essential first step for the well-being of the mother:

> I think that what is required is a home visit by a midwife
> antenatally on diagnosis, to go through all the pros, cons, your
> worries, your fears about the delivery, about what's going to
> happen, how you're going to cope afterwards, the other children,
> the need for rest. I mean, nobody really spelt out to me quite how
> much I ought to have been resting.

Coping

For many mothers there was no time to try and deal with their own
problems and ill health. It was a case of attempting to control their
anxiety about the situation: to attempt to achieve competent control.
In a very different context, Lyng refers to 'the ultimate skill' needed
by individuals who are voluntarily propelled to the limits in search of
themselves: the ability to control a situation that verges on complete
chaos (Lyng 1990).

Descriptions in interviews included attempts to strip away the
responsibility, if only for a matter of moments. Mothers described
such snatched moments: running out of the house to the street corner
and back. Running to the garden shed and back. Locking the children
in one room, leaving the house and crossing the road to the village
shop. These accounts, at first strange, entered into my sense of the
commonplace in this triplet situation. The weight of responsibility
overwhelmed, and culminated in a token physical flight.

One mother of triplets told her health visitor about her inability to
cope:

> I said [to the health visitor] 'I cannot cope, I'm getting to the point
> where something's going to snap, and I don't know what to do.'
> And it took me two or three days to screw up the courage to tell
> her that I couldn't cope with my children. And she said, 'Oh,
> you're being very silly. There's nothing wrong with them. They
> are fit, healthy children and you are coping beautifully. You just
> don't think you're coping.' And then she went away.

The point here is, why is the child-care situation experienced as so
overwhelming? why is there so little provision nation-wide to meet
the mothers' sense of need?

A mother of 3-year-old quadruplets spoke forcefully of how she
tried not to worry:

You know, you reach a point where you no longer worry. You just think 'I cannot worry any more. I'm just going to take things how they come and just muddle through the best I can.' Because that's all one can do. You know, you could easily have a nervous breakdown if you started worrying too much. Even now.

Mothers with triplets, quadruplets or more attract attention. People are curious. Having struggled to get out, mothers reported how they were constantly stopped and questioned by strangers. This is an added pressure:

I am, I suppose, a private person and I have found the amount of attention they attract difficult to cope with. I can't walk down the main street without people approaching me. At times people do, probably unwittingly, make you feel a bit of a freak.

It was difficult enough to maintain the appearance of being in control. Reports of a deceptive 'public' front featured large in interviews. A mother of quintuplets spoke of the front she knew she presented to the world outside her home:

Well, you appear to cope, you see. And if you're organized like I am and you get on with the physical things . . . they're all turned out nicely, they're all behaved on the road because they jolly well had to. We were very strict with them so they [other people] thought, 'Aren't they nice?', 'Isn't she coping well?' And *she* wasn't at all and they didn't see me go home and cry my eyes out and moan at [her husband] and say it's not fair. Nobody knows what it's like.

(Mother's emphasis)

At first, a mother may not even be able to acknowledge to herself her inner turmoil, as one mother of quadruplets pointed out:

[E]verybody thinks – and still thinks – that I coped pretty well and that – you know – I've sailed through it all. Mainly because I wouldn't actually admit for a long time the way [I felt] . . . People were always saying – still now – saying, 'Gosh, you are amazing . . . I don't know how you do it.' Because I have no choice. Absolutely no choice. You either go under a bus, or you cope. One or the other. There is no alternative.

For some an added difficulty was how even to start to express this stress and strain. Some women reported that they were incapable of crying in public. One mother said that she could not cry in such circumstances although she knew that was what was expected of her at meetings with local social services, arranged to discuss whether to continue funding the help she received. 'If you don't cry', she explained, 'people think you are coping'. Nissel and Bonnerjea make a similar observation in relation to women who care for the handicapped elderly:

> Women had to interpret the situation as a crisis to themselves, then they had to present an acceptable definition of a breakdown to the doctor; then help would be provided. One interviewee offered some advice to others in her position: 'You have to be a damn good actress; if you're seen to be coping, you're left alone and there's no help, no share of responsibility. It's very unfair.'
>
> (Nissel and Bonnerjea 1982: 20)

A mother of triplets remarked in interview,

> Until you actually break down in somebody's house and weep all over the place, they're really actually not going to recognize that you've got a need, because they can't understand . . . And I think what I found . . . during the toddler stage particularly – was people just had no idea of what it was like. I mean, you'd recount these dreadful stories of – stories that to you were dreadful, of dreadful days you'd had, and people would think they were terribly funny. And in retrospect they were. But at the time, when they stand in the cat's bowl or eat the cat's food, and they've posted Lego down the toilet, and they've ripped the telephone off the wall, and they've smashed granny's antique vase, then it isn't funny.

Mothers wrote and spoke of the need to get some sleep, and to ensure that their children were fed with the minimum of stress. But some of these children will pose particular difficulties (Chetwynd 1985). Although information from replies to the survey of general practitioners in the National Study had to be interpreted with care because of the poor response, they showed a raised prevalence of cerebral palsy, congenital malformations, pyloric stenosis and hospital admissions among these children (Macfarlane et al. 1990).

Mothers also needed time to themselves away from the continuous care of their children. The difficulties arose when there was uncertainty as to who would provide such help, when, and at what cost. It could not be taken for granted that relatives would rally round (Glendinning 1983; O'Connor and Brown 1984; Hill

1987). Relatives were not always able, or willing, to help, although the majority of mothers in the Parents' Study had at least one relative on whom they had relied for support and practical help in the crucial early months after some or all of their triplets or quadruplets came home from hospital (Price 1990). But few could provide sustained help and support beyond this time. Over half of the parents reported that their relatives had difficulty providing assistance because of their age, infirmity, distance or lack of transport. Not many parents could rely on relatives for long-term help and support on a daily basis. In addition, fewer than half of the parents recorded that they had one or more friend or neighbour who had provided regular support and practical help during the first year. About a third of the parents had no help from relatives, friends or neighbours in the first year after the birth.

The scale of the task of attempting to meet the diverse needs and demands of mothers who were caring for their triplets and higher order multiple birth children, and some of the difficulties of voluntary agency involvement, were evident in the responses to a questionnaire survey of all Home-Start schemes, undertaken by Home-Start Consultancy at my request during the last months of the Parents' Study.

Volunteers from local Home-Start schemes visit and strive to support mothers with children under 5 in their own homes. The co-ordinating body for all the schemes, the Home-Start Consultancy, is a voluntary agency, set up as a partnership between the voluntary and statutory sector (van der Eyken 1982; Gibbons and Thorpe 1989).

In July 1989, 26 out of the 51 Home-Start schemes for which there was a response to the survey reported that they were providing or had provided volunteers for 40 households which included triplets or quads. In addition, two schemes anticipated that they would shortly provide such support. In total, 52 volunteers had been involved, either visiting sequentially – sometimes as many as five volunteers had been involved with one household – or working together in pairs (to provide help with feeding, for instance). Each volunteer provided an average of between 6 and 8 hours per week, although two Home-Start organizers reported that, in cases in which they were involved, volunteers had provided help for 18 and 20 hours per week respectively.

It is difficult to envisage, in the light of the responses to the Home-Start survey, any one volunteer providing more than supplementary or complementary assistance and support over an extended period to mothers in these circumstances. The introduction of many different helpers, however capable and even if provided sequentially, may cause additional stress in the confines of a home. As one Home-Start organizer noted, 'Even coping with an army of different helpers is tiring.'

Conclusion

Not only is the sheer number of same-age children unusual but so too are the cumulative effects of arrangements which have to be made for their care. It takes time to adjust to the magnitude of the responsibilities involved and to the urgent and unfamiliar quest to find others regularly and reliably to assist with tasks through night and day. The analysis of the Parents' Study data left no doubt that it is impossible to cope alone for any length of time.

There are, however, difficulties with local authority provision. We found a marked lack of co-ordination and flexibility with respect to some service provision, leading to a waste of scarce and costly resources: inappropriate people were unreliably provided at the wrong time, to undertake tasks not ranked as a high priority. Difficulties remained unspoken by mothers who feared losing the service.

The professionals themselves were often distressed by the inadequacy of the support they could offer:

> Neither of the two social workers who have dealt with such families recently feel we were able to offer adequate support. Having triplets is quite mind-blowing in terms of demand on parents, emotionally, financially and in every other way. Physical recovery post-delivery takes so much longer. There is no real breathing-space to regain physical fitness. The day-in, day-out pressure of work is exhausting and new pressures arrive at each stage. Both our families have two other children besides and it has not been possible to do any direct work with them.
> (Comment added to UK Social Services Department Survey questionnaire, November 1988)

The identification of budgets to fund service provision to these 'cases' also poses problems. One local authority social services department manager summed it up by saying,

> Such cases do not easily 'fit' in terms of local authority provision
> – i.e. not elderly, not handicapped, no real question of reception
> into care. Require some 'imaginative' and liberal interpretation of
> guide-lines and legislation.

Unless there is some flexibility in the interpretation of guide-lines
mothers may be left feeling bruised and bewildered. There is evidence
of disunity and uncertainty at the administrative level between the
service providers. An evaluation of the power structures behind the
service provision to these mothers would show the extent to which
these structures are in a state of internal tension (Dingwall *et al.* 1983).

One such situation was highlighted by a community nursing
manager in her response to the national survey of community
nursing provision:

> [This Health Authority] had great difficulty getting the Social
> Services Department to understand the real hardships exper-
> ienced by this family by having to deal with triplets as well as
> a four year old sibling. Notice was given to the family that the
> little help they were having would be withdrawn when the triplets
> were one year old. This caused great concern to the Health Visitor
> and communications between Health Visiting and Social Services
> became difficult and strained. At a resulting Case Conference it
> emerged that the reason the Assistant Director gave the mother
> for withdrawing help was that when the children were one year
> old they would become '*easier* to manage'. That statement summed
> up Social Service Department's Assistant Director's degree of
> understanding of children's development, their needs and the
> family's needs. We were able to get them to understand that on
> the contrary the demand would be different but increased. The
> result is Social Services now provide:
>
> Family Aide: four and a half hours a week.
> Home Help: two days a week, 9–11.
> Children's Nanny: Wednesday and Thursday, 11 a.m. to 4
> p.m.
> This family has certainly highlighted for this Health Authority
> the more specific health and emotional needs of such families
> and ways in which we should in the future plan for their care.
> (emphasis in original)

The entry for 27 March 1989 in the diary kept by the mother of the
same triplets reads,

> Discussion with social worker takes place . . . Nothing on earth can describe my anger . . . Actually asked if I wanted the babies taken into care, and offered me counselling for my feelings towards the babies. I just need help with physically caring for them. How dare they treat me like that.

A social worker who was striving to obtain assistance for another mother of triplets summed up the paradox:

> I find it very frustrating in this case that [the mother of triplets] had to be seen to be 'not coping' to justify her need for help and that this is an insistence on looking at her tiredness and anxiety as a medical/psychological problem rather than as a response to the enormous task she is dealing with.

A card arrived in my post one day in August 1990 after the research on which this chapter draws was published. A mother of triplets had written,

> I don't know if you realise what a relief it is to us to have been given the opportunity to speak about the stress we have been under as parents of (naturally conceived) triplets, and how encouraged we are to see the publicity about the plight of multiple families. If nothing else it will raise public awareness. Many of our close friends and contacts have been surprised to learn via the newspapers of the reality we have lived with. I suppose our public front has been a convincing picture of cool, calm, coping people. The truth being much more frenzied!

She echoed a view expressed time and again in the course of the research; the stress of being the mother of triplets, quadruplets and quintuplets was often contained within four walls. It was concealed from others. The impact on health can be profound and impinges on all relationships, complicating mothering. Hilary Graham has observed that successful motherhood is about coping (Graham 1982). To complain is not to cope.

Acknowledgements

Jill Brown, Helen Roberts, Gail Vines and Nina Wakeford each provided vital help and encouragement for which I am very grateful. The Parents' Study could not have been completed without the support of Beverley Botting, Elizabeth Bryan, Alison Macfarlane,

Martin Richards, Sally Roberts and John Wakeford.

The Parents' Study was supported by the Department of Health under its Small Grants Scheme (JS 240/85/13).

References

Botting, B., Macdonald Davies, I., Macfarlane, A. (1987) 'Recent trends in the incidence of multiple births and associated mortality', *Archives of Diseases in Childhood* 62: 941–50.

Botting, B.J., Macfarlane, A. J. and Price, F. V. (1990) *Three, Four or More: A Study of Triplets and Higher Order Births*, London: HMSO.

Bryan, E. (1984) *Twins in the Family: A Parents' Guide*, London: Constable.

Chetwynd, J. (1985) 'Factors contributing to stress on mothers caring for an intellectually handicapped child', *British Journal of Social Work* 15: 295–304.

Dingwall, R., Eekelaar, J. M. and Murray, T. (1983) *The Protection of Children: State Intervention and Family Life*, Oxford, Blackwell.

Gibbons, J. and Thorpe, S. (1989) 'Can voluntary support projects help vulnerable families? The work of Home-Start', *British Journal of Social Work* 19: 189–202.

Glendinning, C. (1983) *Unshared Care: Parents and their Disabled Children*, London: Routledge & Kegan Paul.

Goshen-Gottstein, E. R. (1980) 'The mothering of twins, triplets and quadruplets', *Psychiatry* 43: 189–204.

Graham, H. (1982) 'Coping, or how mothers are seen and not heard', in S. Frudmarsh and E. Sarah (eds) *On the Problems of Men*, London: The Women's Press.

Graham, H. (1984) 'Surveying through stories', in C. Bell and H. Roberts (eds) *Social Researching: Politics, Problems, Practice*, London: Routledge & Kegan Paul.

Haslam, D. R. (1982) 'Sleep loss, recovery sleep, and military performance', *Ergonomics* 25: 163–78.

Hays, P. M. and Smeltzer, J. S. (1986) 'Multiple gestation', *Clinics in Obstetrics and Gynaecology* 29: 264.

Hill, M. (1987) *Sharing Child Care in Early Parenthood*, London: Routledge & Kegan Paul.

Interim Licensing Authority (ILA) (1990) *The Fifth Report of the Interim Licensing Authority for Human In Vitro Fertilisation and Embryology* London: Interim Licensing Authority.

The Lancet (1989), 'The dangers of not going to bed', (editorial) *The Lancet* 1: 138–9.

Lyng, S. (1990) 'Edgework: A social psychological analysis of voluntary risk taking', *American Journal of Sociology* 95: 882–90.

Macfarlane, A. J., Johnson, A., Bower, P. (1990) 'Disabilities and health problems in childhood', in B. J. Botting, A. J. Macfarlane, F. V. Price (eds) *Three, Four and More: A Study of Triplets and Higher Order Births*, London: HMSO.

MacGillivray, I., Campbell, D. M., Thompson, B. (eds) (1988) *Twinning and Twins*, Chichester: John Wiley.

MRC Working Party on Children Conceived by In Vitro Fertilisation (1990) 'Births in Great Britain resulting from assisted conception, 1978–87', *British Medical Journal* 300: 1229–33.

Nissel, M. and Bonnerjea, L. (1982) *Family Care of the Handicapped Elderly: Who Pays?*, London: Policy Studies Institute.

O'Connor, P. D. and Brown, G. W. (1984) 'Supportive relationships: Fact or fancy?', *Journal of Social and Personal Relationships* 1: 159–75.

Orton, D. I. and Gruzelier, J. H. (1989) 'Adverse changes in mood and cognitive performance of house officers after night duty', *British Medical Journal* 298: 21–3.

Patterson, B., Stanley, F. J., Henderson, D. (forthcoming) 'Cerebral palsy in multiple births in Western Australia', *American Journal of Medical Genetics*.

Perridge, T. (1985) *Supertwins Newsletter* 3, London: Twins and Multiple Births Association.

Price, F. V. (1989) *Report to the Parents of Triplets, Quads and Quins*, Cambridge: Child Care and Development Group, University of Cambridge (Crown copyright).

Price, F. V. (1990) 'Who helps?', in B. J. Botting, A. J. Macfarlane, F. V. Price (eds) *Three, Four and More: A Study of Triplets and Higher Order Births*, London: HMSO.

Schenker, J. G., Yarkoni, S., Granat, M. (1981) 'Multiple pregnancies following induction of ovulation', *Fertility and Sterility* 35: 105–23.

Showers, J. and McCleery, J. T. (1984) 'Research on twins: implications for parenting', *Child: Care, Health and Development* 10: 391–404.

Stanley, F. (1984) 'Social and biological determinants of the cerebral palsies', in F. Stanley and E. Alberman (eds) *The Epidemiology of the Cerebral Palsies*, Oxford: Spastics International Medical Publications.

Syrop, C. H. and Varner, M. W. (1985) 'Triplet gestation: maternal and neonatal implications', *Acta Genetica Medica Gemellogica* 34: 81–8.

Topping, K. (1983) *Supertwins Newsletter* 4, London: Twins and Multiple Births Association.

van der Eyken, W. (1982) *Home-Start: A Four Year Evaluation*, Leicester: Home-Start Consultancy.

Willmott, M. (1987) 'Postal surveys of professional groups', SCPR, Survey Methods Newsletter summer: 10–11.

Chapter 8

Working in the dark
Researching female prostitution

Marina Barnard

It is a relatively recent notion in the social sciences that social research is inherently reflexive because it is part of the social world it studies (Schutz 1970; Garfinkel 1967). As such it affects and is affected by the object of its study. This shift in perspective has had the effect of focusing attention upon the means by which data are generated. The methods used to elicit data and the ethics of their use have become increasingly salient concerns for researchers. Once a complex relationship between researcher, research subject and research setting has been acknowledged method cannot be treated simplistically as an unproblematic means to an end. The purpose of this chapter is to look in some detail at the nexus of methodological and ethical issues which arose in the context of a study of female street-working prostitution in Glasgow.

Prostitution as an illegal and stigmatized profession raises particular methodological problems of access and data collection (McLeod 1982) which have become more sharply focused with the advent of HIV and AIDS. A problem for researchers working in this area lies in the ethics of researching a population at risk of a life threatening illness. In this situation, are the researchers justified in providing prostitute women with the means to avoid HIV? Issues of method, access and data collection and also the ethics of studying a population at risk of HIV infection should not be seen as discrete; to an important extent they are overlapping concerns. However, for purposes of clarity they are treated separately in this chapter.

The research described here on prostituting women arose in the context of an ethnographic research project looking in detail at young people's risks of HIV infection through injecting drug use or the practice of unsafe sex. The project is based in an inner-city housing scheme in Glasgow. Three broad groups of people were contacted: injecting drug users in contact with drug treatment agencies, injecting drug users not in contact with treatment agencies, and finally, young people prospectively at risk of drug injecting and HIV infection through living in an area where these conditions are prevalent. The majority of prostituting women described here were contacted in the red light district and were not in contact with drug treatment agencies. However some women were contacted in agency settings such as the city needle exchange and two drug detoxification units. These locations, where relevant, will be indicated after the extracts which follow, which are all taken from my notes.

Prostitution and HIV

The emergent data on prostitution as a potential source of HIV infection is variable. In sub-Saharan Africa prostitution has been clearly associated with the heterosexual spread of HIV (D'Costa *et al*. 1985; Kreiss *et al*. 1986). However there is little similarity between HIV and AIDS data from Africa and from Europe or North America; this suggests that prostitution *per se* is not a significant factor (Day 1988; Cohen 1989). Evidence from the United States shows rates of HIV infection among prostitutes as being proportionate to rates for the total population in each area (MMWR 1987).

However, particular concern has been expressed over injecting drug users who use prostitution as a means of finance. Fears of a heterosexual epidemic of HIV infection have centred on the sexual contacts of those engaging in high risk activities (such as some types of unprotected male homosexual sex or injecting drug use) with the general non-drug-using population (Moss 1987). Certainly the evidence from New York City indicates that heterosexual transmission of the virus is most frequently associated with sexual contact with an injecting drug user (Des Jarlais *et al*. 1987; Stone-burner *et al*. 1990). Injecting drug users (whether male or female) who engage in prostitution to finance their own or their partners' drug use are thus a focus of concern, particularly as raised levels of HIV infection have been identified among this group (MMWR 1987; Tirelli *et al*. 1989). Data from studies in Edinburgh (Morgan Thomas *et al*. 1989), Birmingham (Kinnell 1989) and Manchester (Faugier, personal communication) indicate that significant numbers of women may be prostituting to pay for a drug injecting habit. Our own data from Glasgow show that almost 60 per cent of those street-working prostitute women contacted were themselves injecting drug users (McKeganey *et al*. 1990a). These women may be doubly at risk of HIV infection through injecting drug use and sexual transmission.

Notwithstanding this, prostitution does not currently look set to play a pivotal role in the widespread transmission of HIV infection, for two reasons. First, research on prostitutes suggests that insistence on client condom use by female prostitutes is widespread (Day *et al*. 1988; McKeganey *et al*. 1990a), and is motivated by a concern to protect both themselves and their clients from HIV infection. Second, recent epidemiological evidence from the developed world indicates that male to female heterosexual transmission of the virus is more likely than from female to male (Padian 1988; Stoneburner *et al*. 1990). Thus it may be that female prostitutes are at greater risk from their clients than their clients are from them.

Locating prostituting women

Contacting women who prostituted was one of the study objectives. However, we encountered a reluctance amongst women living in the study area to volunteer information on the use of prostitution as a means of finance. This raised problems of locating and contacting prostitute women in sufficient numbers for the purposes of research. We were reluctant to negotiate access to service environments, such as sexually transmitted diseases clinics, in the hope of contacting prostitute women because it is known that many women who engage in a drug injecting life-style make uneven and inconsistent use of services. Successful contact in such an environment would depend on the woman identifying herself as working as a prostitute. It is understandable that she might want to avoid this. The following field extract illustrates the reticence encountered in women in research locations other than the red light area in providing information on the use of prostitution as a means of financing a drug habit:

> I had a feeling she might be working in the town because she said she was injecting heroin 4 times a day and she'd never been in the jail (except once for 3 days) in all the time she'd been injecting, so it seemed likely she wasn't shoplifting. So I asked her if she wanted condoms. She said 'Aye' and I asked her if she wanted the tasteless ones (these are used for the provision of oral sex to clients) which she said yes to. So then I felt I could ask if she was working in the town and she said she was. I said she might see me down there in the near future but that she wasn't to worry, that I wasn't part of

the needle exchange and I had no note of her name. 'I don't want ma name on anythin'' she said firmly in reply.

(Needle Exchange)

We encountered a general reluctance among the young people we were in contact with to discuss the subject of sex and sexuality. Where it was raised it frequently met with embarrassment and awkwardness (Barnard and McKeganey 1990), which was often sufficient to foreclose discussion relating specifically to prostitution.

To counter problems of access and identification it was decided that the best means of contacting women in sufficient numbers was to carry out research in the red light district. Fieldwork was done by a female and a male researcher. However contact was initiated and sustained primarily by the female (myself), as approach by the male researcher in this context was likely to be misinterpreted by the prostitutes. We time-sampled across each day of the week and across each of the time periods the women worked. We aimed to look in detail at HIV risk related activities, such as injecting drugs and the provision of unsafe sex, and the risk reduction strategies, if any, adopted by prostitute women. Additionally, we wanted to develop some means of assessing the numbers of Glasgow street-working prostitutes who injected drugs and those who did not.

Contacting prostituting women

It is one thing to locate a study population, it is quite another to initiate the type of contact which enables the development of a good enough research relationship to collect what is often sensitive and personal data. From this perspective an important dimension to our contact with prostituting women was the incorporation of a service provider role into the research process. All the women we contacted were offered condoms or sterile injecting equipment, or both, as well as an advice leaflet detailing contact addresses of various voluntary and statutory helping agencies. The inclusion of service provision into the research facilitated contact and helped provide the women with a plausible explanation for our continued presence in the area.

The red light district is unambiguously concerned with the buying and selling of sexual services which puts clear limits on the range of reasons for lingering in the area. Many of the women were quite justifiably suspicious, and on some occasions hostile towards people whose motivations were not clearly understood. Women engaging in prostitution have to be constantly vigilant, both of police activity and of dangerous clients. Many women have children and fear the consequences of identification as a prostitute by the statutory agencies. Few women who prostitute can be unaware of, or immune to, the adverse comment which attaches to prostitution. A woman described the experience of working as a prostitute:-

> Working on the streets puts a lot of pressure on your mind because of what you're doin'. I got in trouble with the vice but it wasn't that so much as what I was doin' for money. A lot of times I'd hit before I went to ma work so I didnae think about it, and then after I left ma work I had a hit.
>
> (Drug Detoxification Unit)

Women were wary of us if they thought we were plain clothes police. Quickly establishing that we had no connection with the police or the statutory agencies was therefore important, as was making clear our purpose as researchers. The following field extract illustrates the women's frequent identification of us as police ('the vice') at least in the early days of the research:

> Last night at about midnight we saw a girl who was clearly working. I began walking over to her and she immediately walked off really quickly. I called over to her but she didn't stop. Finally I said 'Look I'm not police or anything'. She stopped then, clearly afraid. I gave her needles and syringes and condoms. She was just starting work and was looking for someone to give her condoms because she didn't have any.

Subsequent meetings with this woman were not problematic, presumably because she no longer construed our presence as a threat to her. What we were not (police, social workers) was apparently of greater importance than what we were (researchers). The relevant and important issue for the women seemed to be the clear establishment by the researcher of 'good intention' (Johnson 1975). This at least was our impression:

> Neil and I have been going around the red light district for just over a week now. At first when we approached the women they were reticent and clearly wondered who we were. Some women seemed reluctant to say they were injecting drugs even though we felt they probably were. However we have now spoken to about seventy women and word has spread. They don't seem entirely

sure of what it is we do, describing us in vague terms like, 'fae the university'. They don't seem to regard us as doing them any harm.

As Wax (1971) and Whyte (1943) have indicated, the good will of research subjects appears more dependent upon a positive assessment of the researcher in personal terms than upon agreement with, or even interest in, the research objectives.

The research bargain

The provision of condoms or sterile injecting equipment undoubtedly facilitated the initiation and continuation of contact between ourselves and the women working as prostitutes. Many of the women appeared to believe that this was our main, if not sole, reason for being there:

> We approached a woman new to us. She identified us with 'you's the one's doin' tools [injecting equipment]? Gonnae gie us a set? I've been tryin' to find youse for ages but I didnae know what you looked like.'

As far as the women were concerned, the services we provided in large part explained our presence in the red light district over many months; for us service provision played an important part in facilitating contact with the women. Similar research bargains are reported to have been struck, particularly in research work with deviant groups such as drug users (Carey 1972).

The prominence given by the women to the service dimension of our work may have been influenced by the fact that they saw no evidence of the obvious tools of the researcher's trade, such as the ubiquitous questionnaire. Given the research setting and the limited time women were willing or able to make available, there was no scope for the use of a questionnaire. The preferred strategy was to collect data informally through brief but consistent contact with the women and as systematically as possible to build up a detailed understanding of the work they did as prostitutes. The provision of services that were valued by the women played an important facilitating role in the successful maintenance of this research strategy. The provision of either needles or condoms could itself be a source of data:

> When we have given out needles, women have often expressed relief because something has happened to render theirs useless.

'Oh thank God, mines have just snapped . . . let me tell you what happened just now' . . . On at least three occasions women have said that their works were no good and have taken new ones from us. The majority of women seem to use the small 1 ml syringes yet they seem the most vulnerable. When they break what do the women do? In that area at night there isn't any means of getting clean needles, so do they share in those circumstances?

Identifying drug using prostitutes

One of the objectives of this research was to calculate the prevalence of street-working prostitution in Glasgow and the proportion of prostituting women who were injecting drug users relative to those who were not. The method used to model the prevalence of prostituting women working the streets is described elsewhere (McKeganey *et al.* 1990b). Here we are concerned with the problem of distinguishing prostitute women who inject drugs from those who do not.

Rather than relying on the women to self-report injecting drug use, all the women contacted were offered sterile injecting equipment. This was an important means by which women who were injecting drug users could be distinguished from those who were not. Where a woman did take injecting equipment, supplementary information was sought in an effort to confirm that it was indeed she who was injecting and not someone else. Confirmatory evidence of drug use most often centred on knowledge of drugs, needle and syringe types, and drug experiences. We found the display of this type of knowledge a fairly reliable indicator of personal drug use. Through this method it was ascertained that 59 per cent of all streetworking women contacted were injecting drug users (McKeganey *et al.* 1990a).

The advent of a new and life threatening disease has placed a premium on researchers gaining access to populations generally recognized as difficult to contact and research. In our experience the successful resolution of issues of access and sustained contact with these populations was in large part due to the adoption of a flexible and pragmatic research design, one, in Leviton's words, 'specifically targetted to the circumstances' (1989: 42). In these terms the incorporation of service provision into the research proved a successful strategy.

Researching prostitution: ethical issues

Two interrelated issues concerning the ethics of service provision can be identified here. First, does providing injecting equipment condone injecting drug use? Since HIV infection is known to be transmitted through the use of unsterile needles and syringes is it acceptable to withhold from drug injectors the means to minimize their risks of infection? Second, in research terms, is it good scientific practice for the researcher to incorporate the role of service provider within the research role? In providing the women with the means to reduce their risks of HIV infection the researcher clearly has an effect upon the risk practices that are to be studied. Additionally, because the role of service provider is a more familiar and better understood role than that of researcher, the research role may be viewed as inconsequential by the respondent, even though it is the prime reason for contact in the mind of the researcher. Thus whilst the researcher might feel she has made clear her purpose, a certain blurring of the edges is bound to occur over time where the two roles are interwoven. The question then is whether or not the research can be said to have the informed consent of its subjects where contact is sustained largely through means of providing a service useful to the women.

The ethics of providing the means to inject drugs

In the context of the establishment of syringe exchange schemes in England and Scotland since 1987, the debate concerning the ethics of providing drug injectors with sterile injecting equipment has been heated (Stimson *et al.* 1988). Practitioners in the field of drug addiction tend to fall into two broad camps: there are those who advocate complete abstinence from drugs and those who favour a gradual withdrawal (Stimson 1989). Those in the former camp argue that for health practitioners to provide the means to inject is a contradictory practice and does nothing to encourage the cessation of drug use (Farid 1988). Those more disposed towards harm reduction generally argue that abstinence, although a laudable goal, is not attainable by some drug injectors (Robertson *et al.* 1986). Thus if some drug injectors cannot, or will not stop injecting, they can at least be provided with the means to prevent cross-infection through sharing unsterile needles and syringes. This argument is particularly salient in the light of the apparent connection between non-availability of sterile injecting equipment in Edinburgh and the epidemic spread of HIV among drug injectors (SHHD 1986; Robertson 1990).

The adoption of a more pragmatic public health position has resulted in increased availability of clean injecting equipment to prevent spread of HIV infection. From this perspective, our provision of needles and syringes to those considered at risk of HIV infection is in line with current public health thinking in the UK. As part of a harm reduction strategy we considered this an ethical practice.

The main red light district is located in a primarily commercial part of the city. Few shops are open at night and certainly there is no chemist selling injecting equipment. Drug injectors accept that in the normal run of things needles break or become blunt and syringes block, rendering equipment useless. If this happens a woman may feel she has no choice but to use someone else's equipment to inject with. Instances of women asking to make use of another's injecting equipment were commonly reported:

> We stood talking to two women, one mentioned needle sharing, 'aye, like that lassie the other night goin' round askin' everyone if they'd lend her a set. She even asked me, and I'm a stranger, she was askin' everyone, She could've used someone's that's got AIDS.'

In the face of the risks attached to using someone else's needle and syringe it might seem a more sensible response for the woman to forego injecting altogether. However so far as the women were concerned this was not a viable option. There are two main reasons for this: first, in foregoing injection of drugs a woman faces the sure prospect of very unpleasant withdrawal symptoms. Second, whilst the majority of prostitute women who injected drugs represented prostitution as a necessary evil to fund an expensive habit they reported their work impossible without drugs to numb the experience:

> Sally described prostitution as 'quick money but no easy money, your head's wasted with it. That's what used to stop me from working 'cos ma head was all done in. I could never work straight. I'd need to have somethin' in me even if I didnae have a habit.'
> (Drug Detoxification Unit)

There remains the unresolved dilemma that increasing needle and syringe availability could result in spreading the virus, because individuals might be encouraged to begin drug injecting as a consequence (Cook 1987; Farid 1988). The researchers were aware of this possibility and would not knowingly have supplied a potential initiate with injecting equipment. However, framing the response to this dilemma in terms of the researchers' knowledge and good intentions sidesteps the issue of responsibility. The possibility exists that in making needles and syringes available, we have inadvertently facilitated a woman's induction (or reintroduction) into injecting drug use.

Deciding whether or not to supply the women with injecting equipment had consequences either way. On the one hand there is the apparent condoning of a dangerous and illegal habit through providing the means to inject and potentially, if not intentionally, being responsible for a woman's induction into injecting drug use. On the other hand the free provision of a scarce commodity was valued by the women as a practical means to reduce their risks of infection. The issue was not clear cut, and some responsibility for any negative consequences of either course of action would have to be borne by the researchers.

The ethics of an incorporating service provision into a research role

From our perspective, and that of others (Schutz 1970; Emerson 1981; Hammersley and Atkinson 1983), research in the social sciences is by its very nature an interactive process. Whatever the method used the researcher cannot be erased from the research equation. Gender, class, ethnicity and personality all shape the quality of the interaction and influence the data collected as well as its subsequent interpretation (Easterday et al. 1977; Stanley and Wise 1983; Jenkins 1984; McKeganey and Bloor 1991). From this perspective the issue was whether a research role that incorporated a service provider role would be to the detriment of the research objectives. For instance, it was possible that the women might be reluctant to report risk practices to us because we were supplying them with the means to avoid them. To report risk behaviour as ongoing might in the eyes of some of the women jeopardize our good will and most important, the continued supply of needles and syringes. As Johnson argues, knowledge is never neutral and should be viewed as 'use oriented, as being related to the personal interests and practical purposes of the knower' (1975: 133).

The first point to note is that information management should be seen as an integral feature of all social interaction and certainly not unique to the situation described here. Our data indicate that the women were managing information, not only in their relations with us, but also with other prostituting women. The fact that we provided needles and syringes may have resulted in some under-reporting of risk behaviours. However women did comment on their own risk behaviour, often in a very unselfconscious manner, which suggested to us that they did not see the supply of either condoms or injecting equipment as conditional upon our favourable assessment of their efforts to reduce risk taking behaviour:

> A woman we had just given a needle and syringe to asked for another set for her boyfriend. I said that her set had been the last of them. 'Oh well then' she said, 'it doesnae matter, we'll just use the one set.'

The second point to note is that seeking to control the flow of certain types of information both to us and amongst themselves was itself a source of illuminating data, revealing the operation of a 'code of practice' amongst female street-working prostitutes. Certain types of behaviour were clearly considered unacceptable. These principally concerned undercutting an accepted price structure for sexual practices and not using a condom with a client. Also (although to a much lesser degree), the sharing of unsterile injecting equipment was perceived negatively by the women. Thus although we estimate that we spoke to approximately two-thirds of the women prostituting on the streets, none reported that she had infringed the first two of these norms, although there were frequently cited instances of other women having done so:

> Susan said she was often asked by clients to agree to sex without a condom and if you refused, the guy would drive off and later on you'd see a girl getting into the car and you'd know then that she was doing it without a condom. She spoke of a girl 'doin' it for fivers without a condom, anything. The girls were cracking up over it, we told her but she didnae take any notice, so finally we told the vice and the vice then drove her out of this town saying to her "if you're going to work at all, you should work properly".'

and:

> I asked if she got asked for sex without a condom, 'Aye a lot, last night I got asked but I just say get t'fuck, I'm no' doin' it without a condom. She then added that the client would just ask somebody else 'They keep askin' until they get one that'll do it without one.'

It is probable that certain types of information were withheld from the researchers. The degree to which this was as a specific consequence of the inclusion of a service provider role is difficult to judge. Whilst service provision facilitated access and was a useful means of focusing on the research concerns, it may also have placed constraints on the information women were willing to impart. However, information which the women sought to manage was itself revealing and hence of benefit to the research.

An important tenet of good sociological practice is that researchers should have the informed consent of the research participants (British Sociological Association 1973). In brief, informed consent relates to the ethical responsibility of a researcher to explain fully what the purpose of the research is, who is doing it, who it is funded by and why it is being done. With this information the research respondent can make an informed choice as to whether or not she or he will agree to be involved in the research.

In the context of this study, however, informed consent was not a straightforward and uncomplicated affair. It was problematic in two ways; the first specifically concerns the inclusion of service provision within the research, the second is more generally related to the dynamics of qualitative field research.

The point has been made that many of the prostitute women contacted characterized us primarily as service providers rather than as researchers. The value they attached to the service and the fact that the role of service provider, so far as the women were concerned, better explained our presence perhaps accounts for the overshadowing of the research role. None the less this characterization persisted even though on initial contact we introduced ourselves as researchers, showed an identification card and explained the study and what we were doing. This meant that the women provided us with information on their risk practices and so on, but we were uncertain in some cases whether or not they were aware that we would make notes on what was said.

The research was not covert yet it developed an ambiguous status because of the prominence attributed to service provision. This ambiguity could perhaps have been resolved through regular reiteration of the research project's objectives and our purposes as researchers. There is however a limit to how many times one can repeat the same information without risking the good will of the research subject. As researchers we were not prepared to jeopardize our work by repeatedly insisting on our identity. We had therefore to accept that at least some of the women in seeing us primarily, or only, as service providers did not have a clear sense of the research they were contributing to.

Service provision was not the only factor which influenced the clarity with which the women perceived our role as researchers. Other factors were influential and related to the research setting and also the very nature of qualitative research work.

To a large degree it was the research setting which dictated the use of a qualitative research methodology. There was neither the time nor the place for the use of questionnaires and the like, hence data were collected informally and through observation. We could not take notes openly for fear that this would be ominously interpreted by people who had a vested interest in the women, such as drug dealers and the few pimps in the area. The intention was not to hoodwink the women by recording information out of their sight. It was done out of a sense of regard for our own safety.

Collecting data by way of informal interviewing and observation clearly did little to remove any existing ambiguity over the nature of the research role. Yet it is difficult to see how ambiguity could be avoided, since qualitative methodologies rely heavily upon good interpersonal relationships in order to obtain data on the processes and dynamics of social interaction within and between groups. Developing good relationships implies a process whereby the social distance between those concerned is progressively reduced. However, frequent reiteration of one's research purposes reasserts the distance between researcher and researched and in so doing gives the lie to the social relations one is trying to develop. In trading on personal relationships it is not easy for the researcher to avoid blurring the distinction between personal and professional roles.

Service provision may have hampered the women's perception of ourselves as researchers but other factors were also influential. However, irrespective of the way in which the women perceived us they entrusted us with information about their lives which was often sensitive and could have been used to their detriment. Our position then was one of having an ethical responsibility towards these data such that the women would not be adversely affected by their collection or publication. The stigmatized and relatively powerless position of prostitute women serves only to further underline this responsibility.

The starting point for this discussion was that research as an interactive and creative process involves a constant dialogue between researchers and respondents, which inevitably affects the plan and practice of the research. To illustrate this dialetic between researcher and respondent some of the methodological and ethical issues in the context of the study of prostitution were focused upon. These issues should be seen not as discrete, but as interrelated. In addressing the methodological imperative the ethics of the research also become salient and in need of attention.

For the purpose of this study the research role incorporated a service provider role, the benefits of which were considered to outweigh the costs both in terms of providing a service to the women and achieving the research objectives. Although research was facilitated through providing the women with a service, it was in no sense subordinated to it.

There cannot be a blueprint research design which addresses the full range of methodological and ethical issues raised by the practice of research. Each research project produces a unique constellation of concerns relating specifically to the purposes of the research and the population to be studied. These issues seem best addressed through a judicious mix of pragmatism and flexibility and a concern not only for the best interests of the research but also the researched.

Acknowledgement

I would like to thank Neil McKeganey and Mick Bloor for their insightful comments on an earlier version of this chapter and Margaret Seaforth for typing this manuscript.

Notes

This research is funded by the Economic and Social Research Council and is being conducted by Neil McKeganey and myself. The research into female (and male) prostitution was jointly conducted between ourselves and Michael Bloor, who is employed at the Medical Research Council, Medical Sociology Unit, Glasgow.

The Public Health Research Unit is supported by the Chief Scientist

Office, Scottish Home and Health Department and the Greater Glasgow Health Board. The opinions expressed in this paper are not necessarily those of the Scottish Home and Health Department.

References

Barnard, M.A. and McKeganey, N.P. (1990) 'Adolescents and injecting drug use; Risks for HIV infection', *AIDS Care* 2(2): 106–16.

British Sociological Association (1973) *Statement of Ethical Principles and their Application to Sociological Practice* (under revision), London: BSA.

Carey, J.T. (1972) 'Problems of access and risk in observing drug scenes', in J.D. Douglas (ed.) *Research on Deviance*, New York: Basic Books, 71–89.

Cohen, J.B. (1989) 'Overstating the risk of AIDS: Scapegoating prostitutes', *Focus, a Guide to AIDS Research* 4(2): 1–2.

Cook, C.C.H. (1987) 'Syringe exchange 1', *The Lancet* 1: 920–21.

Day, S. (1988) 'Prostitute women and AIDS: Anthropology', *AIDS* 2: 421–8.

Day, S., Ward, H., Harris, J.R.W. (1988) 'Prostitute women and public health', *British Medical Journal* 297: 1585.

D'Costa, L.J., Plummer, F.A., Bowner, J. *et al.* (1985) 'Prostitutes are a major reservoir of transmitted diseases in Nairobi, Kenya', *Sexually Transmitted Diseases* 12: 64–7.

Des Jarlais, D.C., Wish, E., Friedman, S.R., Stoneburner, R. *et al.* (1987) 'Intravenous drug use and the heterosexual transmission of the Human Immunodeficiency Virus: Current trends in New York City', *New York State Journal of Medicine* May: 283–6.

Easterday, L., Papademas, D., Schoor, L., Valentine, C. (1977) 'The making of a female researcher', *Urban Life* 6: 333–49.

Emerson, R.M. (1981) 'Observational fieldwork', *Annual Review of Sociology* 7: 351–78.

Farid, B.T. (1988) 'AIDS and drug addiction needle exchange schemes: A step in the dark', *Journal of the Royal Society of Medicine* 81: 375–6.

Garfinkel, H. (1967) *Studies in Ethnomethodology*, Englewood Cliffs, NJ: Prentice Hall.

Hammersley, M. and Atkinson, P. (1983) *Ethnography: Principles in Practice*, London: Tavistock.

Jenkins, R. (1984) 'Bringing it all back home: An anthropologist in Belfast', in C. Bell and H. Roberts (eds) *Social Researching: Politics, Problems, Practice*, London: Routledge & Kegan Paul, 147–64.

Johnson. J.M. (1975) *Doing Field Research*, New York: The Free Press.

Kinnell, H. (1989) *Prostitutes, Their Clients and Risks of HIV Infection in Birmingham*, Occasional paper, Birmingham: Department of Public Health Medicine.

Kreiss, J. K., Koech, D., Plummer, F. A. *et al.* (1986) 'AIDS virus infection in Nairobi prostitutes: spread of the epidemic to East Africa', *New England Journal of Medicine* 314: 414–18.

Leviton, L. C. (1989) 'Theoretical foundations of AIDS-Prevention Programs', in R. O. Valdiserri (ed.) *Preventing AIDS: The Design of Effective Programs*, New Brunswick, NJ: Rutgers University Press.

McKeganey, N. P. and Bloor, M. J. (1991) 'Spotting the invisible male: The influence of male gender on fieldwork relations', *British Journal of Sociology* 42(2): 195–210.

McKeganey, N. P., Barnard, M. A., Bloor, M. J. (1990a) 'A comparison of HIV related risk behaviour and risk reduction between female street-working prostitutes and male rent boys in Glasgow', *Sociology of Health and Illness* 12(3): 274–92.

McKeganey, N. P., Barnard, M. A., Bloor, M. J., Leyland, A. (1990b) 'Injecting drug use and female streetworking prostitutes in Glasgow', *AIDS* 4(11): 1153–5.

McLeod, E. (1982) *Women Working: Prostitution Now*, London: Croom Helm.

MMWR, Morbidity and Mortality Weekly Report (1987) Centers for Disease Control, 36: 11.

Morgan Thomas, R., Plant, M. A., Plant M. L., Sales, D. L. (1989) 'Risk of AIDS among workers in the sex industry: Some initial results from a Scottish study', *British Medical Journal* 299: 148–9.

Moss, A. R. (1987) 'AIDS and intravenous drug use: The real heterosexual epidemic', *British Medical Journal* 294: 389–90.

Padian, N. S. (1988) 'Prostitute women and AIDS: Epidemiology', *AIDS* 6: 413–19.

Robertson, R. (1990) 'The Edinburgh epidemic', in J. Strang and G. V. Stimson (eds) *AIDS and Drug Misuse: Understanding and Responding to the Drug Taker in the Wake of HIV*, London: Tavistock.

Robertson, R., Bucknall, A. B. V., Welsby, P. D., Roberts, J. J. K. *et al.* (1986) 'Epidemic of AIDS related virus (HTLV III/LAV) infection among intravenous drug abusers', *British Medical Journal* 292: 527–9.

Schutz, A. (1970) *Reflections on the Problem of Relevance*, New Haven, Conn.: Yale University Press.

Scottish Home and Health Department (1986) *HIV Infection in Scotland: Report of the Scottish Committee on HIV Infection and Intravenous Drug Misuse* Edinburgh: SHHD.

Stanley L., Wise, S., (1983) *Breaking Out: Feminist Consciousness and Feminist Research*, London: Routledge & Kegan Paul.

Stimson, G. V. (1989) 'Editorial review: Syringe exchange programmes for injecting drug users', *AIDS* 3: 253–60.

Stimson, G. V., Donoghoe, M., Aldritt, L., Dolan, K. (1988) 'HIV transmission risk behaviour of clients attending syringe-exchange schemes in England and Scotland', *British Journal of Addiction* 83: 1449–55.

Stoneburner, R., Chaisson, M. A., Weifuse, I., Thomas, P. A. *et al.* (1990) 'The epidemic of AIDS and HIV infection among heterosexuals in New York City', *AIDS* 4(2): 99–106.

Tirelli U., Rezza, G., Guiliani, M., Caprilli, F. *et al.* (1989) 'HIV sero-prevalence among 304 female prostitutes from four Italian towns', *AIDS* 3: 547–8.

Wax, R. (1971) *Doing Fieldwork*, Chicago: University of Chicago Press.

Whyte, W. (1943) *Street Corner Society: the Social Structure of an Italian Slum*, Chicago: University of Chicago Press.

Chapter 9

Research and audit
Women's views of caesarean section

Edith M. Hillan

Increasingly it is recognized that audit should be an integral part of all health care practice. This is one of the seven key changes proposed in the government white paper *Working for Patients* (HMSO 1989).

Audit of perinatal practice has been defined as comprising

> any evaluative process which explicitly aims to provide information which can lead to improvements in the care available to childbearing women and their families. Implicit in common usage of the word 'audit' is that it is a formal process.
>
> (Chalmers 1980)

Until recently there has been a tendency in perinatal care to evaluate any new procedures or practices purely on the grounds of their clinical merit. However, it is increasingly recognized that the social and psychological impact of a new technique on a woman may affect its overall value.

Childbirth is a social and personal experience as well as an obstetric event, and for most women a satisfactory outcome of pregnancy involves more than the delivery of a healthy baby. Few women today view pregnancy and delivery as a series of biological events over which they have no control, and increasingly, they are demanding a more humanistic approach to obstetric care and a greater share of responsibility in decision making related to the care that they receive.

The direct contact which nurses and midwives have with patients means that they can seize the opportunity to develop some aspects of audit, and ensure that it does not merely develop as an exercise in 'counting' but takes into account some of the more subtle processes involved in being a patient. This chapter describes one such project, which was based on caesarean section in a Scottish maternity hospital. Although the nature and extent of this project may be beyond the range of student practitioners including audit and research in their work, it suggests ways in which questions of audit may be broadened out to look at issues of overall satisfaction of women with the care they receive before, during and after childbirth, and the ways in which the findings of research may be incorporated into practice at local level.

The incidence of caesarean section has risen steadily in most developed countries over the last decade. Professional and lay concern about the increase has prompted national reviews in an effort to elicit the reasons for this upward trend (Rosen 1981; Boyd et al. 1983). The most dramatic increase in rates has occurred in the United States, where caesarean births have more than quadrupled: from 5.5 per cent of all deliveries in 1970 (Placek and Taffel 1980) to 24.1 per cent in 1986 (Placek et al. 1988). Although the incidence of caesarean section is lower in Scotland than the USA, the upward trend in the rate is still marked: from 4.2 per cent in 1970 (McIlwaine et al. 1985) to 13.6 per cent in 1987 (Information and Statistics Division 1989).

The claim that there is a direct causal relationship between the fall in perinatal mortality and the rise in the number of caesarean sections being performed is difficult to sustain in the light of evidence from the Netherlands (Thiery and Derom 1986a; 1986b) and a regional hospital in Dublin (O'Driscoll and Foley 1983), where despite stable caesarean section rates the perinatal outcome has improved to the same degree as in countries where caesarean rates have increased.

The clinical indications mainly responsible for the rise in rates are now well described (Rosen 1981) and include dystocia, previous caesarean section, breech presentation and fetal distress. However, there is a lack of evidence to support the use of abdominal delivery for many of these common indications, which led one obstetrician to comment that the increasing caesarean section rate 'is the result of one of the least controlled clinical experiments that has occurred in medicine' (Pearson 1984).

Few studies have addressed the importance of non-clinical variables in decisions to deliver by caesarean section. In the United States, failure to perform a caesarean section is one of the commonest reasons for litigation (Raines 1984) and although malpractice suits are much less common in the United Kingdom, fear of litigation was the second most common reason for performing sections given by British obstetricians in a survey carried out by the Maternity Alliance (Boyd *et al.* 1983).

Although caesarean delivery is now safer than it has ever been, it remains a major surgical procedure and therefore can never be an entirely safe alternative to vaginal delivery. The National Institute of Health Task Force report (Rosen 1981) estimated that the maternal mortality associated with caesarean section was four times greater than that associated with vaginal delivery, and maternal morbidity rates were also greatly increased when delivery was effected by the abdominal route. However, definitions of morbidity lack uniformity and this in turn makes the classification of major and minor complications difficult, so any comparison of morbidity rates is of dubious value. Nevertheless there can be no doubt that morbidity is greater after caesarean delivery than after vaginal delivery.

During the time period in which caesarean section rates have been rising, women's expectations about childbirth have also altered. Factors such as prepared childbirth, paternal participation in labour and delivery, and emphasis on 'gentle birth' and early parent–infant contact for bonding have all contributed to a revolution in attitudes for many parents today (Rosen 1981). Research evidence about the psychological or emotional impact of abdominal delivery on the mother, father and the family unit is fragmentary and preliminary at best.

A number of negative responses to a caesarean delivery among women have been reported (Marut and Mercer 1979; Affonso and Stichler 1980; Cranley *et al.* 1983). These responses include fear, disappointment, anger and lowered self-esteem. In part these reactions may reflect the disparity between prior expectations of the birth and the actual experience, or they may represent a reaction to the presence of complications or a crisis which made the section necessary.

Pregnancy, childbirth and parenthood require massive physiological and psychological adjustments on the part of the woman. Even under normal circumstances the transition to motherhood may be problematical, especially if reality does not meet up with the woman's prior expectations of her delivery. Oakley (1980) found that the most normal of births can involve elements of loss for the mother: loss of self-confidence, loss of body image, loss of previous employment and so on. She states that,

Childbirth is a life event with considerable loss and uncertain gain. The response is liable to be hopelessness and the extent of this is determined in large part by the extent to which people feel able to take control over their own lives.

In addition to these 'normal' stressors, the woman who has had a caesarean section has to cope with the physical and psychological impact of anaesthesia and major surgery, which may have occurred on top of a long and exhausting labour.

Oakley (1983) has commented on the way that caesarean section is conceptualized differently from other types of abdominal surgery. The term section is used as opposed to 'surgery' or 'operation' and this is associated with a difference in the way in which the effects of caesarean section and other surgical procedures are seen. A common, generally accepted consequence of major surgery is depression, yet the same assumption is not made about caesarean section. Similarly, many of the general after-effects of surgery are applicable to caesarean section. These may include a temporary response of emotional relief and elation from having recovered from the anaesthetic, worry about the mutilating effects of the surgery and an extended period of physical and psychological discomfort (Janis 1958). In addition, the woman who has experienced caesarean delivery is often expected to cope with the demands of her new baby, and this may involve activities that are normally forbidden to patients who have undergone abdominal surgery.

Comparatively few studies to date have attempted to evaluate the psychological and social impact of caesarean delivery and those that have are mainly from the USA and Canada and are primarily descriptive in nature. Many of the studies have used non-representative samples, for example parents who voluntarily contacted the researchers or participants in caesarean support groups, and involve small numbers of women. Caesarean support groups offer psychological and social support for women who have experienced caesarean delivery and their numbers have grown rapidly in the USA and to a lesser extent in the United Kingdom. One interesting aspect of these groups is that they have voiced little criticism about the rising caesarean section rates, which implies that the recipients of such surgery tend to view it as being 'necessary'.

Methodology

Many studies have been published on the determinants of the rise in caesarean section rates but comparatively few have addressed the physical, psychological and social consequences for the woman and her baby. So the current study was designed to provide further knowledge of some of the immediate, short-term and longer-term consequences of caesarean section for both the mother and her infant. A study group of fifty low-risk primigravidae (first time mothers) of normal stature delivered by emergency caesarean section was compared with a closely matched control group of fifty primigravidae delivered vaginally.

Data for the study was collected from four sources:

1 The obstetric case record and midwifery notes;
2 A semi-structured hospital interview conducted on the fourth or fifth postnatal day;
3 A postal questionnaire sent out three months after delivery;
4 A semi-structured home interview conducted six months after delivery.

The obstetric case record and midwifery notes provided routine family data about the woman as well as details of the labour, including the reasons for the performance of any operative interventions. Morbidity which developed in the postnatal period was noted, as well as variables such as length of stay in hospital, type of infant feeding and the reported results of any postnatal pelvimetry. The neonatal outcome was documented and included information such as: Apgar scores at one and five minutes; resuscitation methods employed; birth-weight and discharge of the infant from theatre.

The method used for the hospital interview on the fourth or fifth postnatal day was a semi-structured questionnaire. Where appropriate the fifty women in each group were asked the same questions. However, the questionnaire differed slightly for the study and control groups to account for the differing delivery experiences of the women. The hospital interview provided data on sources of information about pregnancy, labour and delivery; the women's feelings about the labour and delivery experience on this occasion; problems experienced since delivery and infant feeding practices.

The postal questionnaire at three months after delivery was intended to determine the short-term morbidity associated with the different delivery methods. On completion it showed the health of women and their babies following discharge from hospital and described the reported morbidity. It also determined the women's knowledge of the reasons for her operative delivery and elicited infant feeding practices. The response rate to the postal questionnaire was 91 per cent.

Permission was also sought at the time of recruitment into the study to contact the women at home six months after delivery in order to conduct a semi-structured face-to-face interview. The purpose of this home interview was to compare the long-term morbidity in the women delivered by caesarean section with those delivered vaginally and to elicit women's views of their labour and delivery experience; their views on future pregnancies; sexual difficulties since delivery and infant health and feeding practices since discharge. Eighty-four per cent of the women delivered by section and 88 per cent of the control group were successfully contacted at this time.

The study generated a large amount of both quantitative and qualitative data. It is not possible to present all of the results within this chapter but some of the comments made by the women about both midwifery and obstetric care are discussed below.

Results

One problem in trying to measure satisfaction with maternity care is that no standardized or validated scales exist for doing so. Just as the recipients of perinatal care are not a homogeneous group, satisfaction will inevitably mean different things to different women. Satisfaction may also be dependent on a number of other factors, including a mother's personality, the amount of preparation received before delivery, prior expectations of childbirth, past childbirth experience, the type of delivery and the degree of control a woman feels she has over her experience. A further difficulty in assessing satisfaction is that it is unstable and changes according to unrelated variables such as the woman's mood at the time of the interview, who is asking the questions, how the questions are posed and how much time has elapsed since the event (Shearer 1983).

Perhaps the greatest difficulty in assessing women's attitudes to caesarean delivery is that few women doubt that the operation is only carried out in cases of 'real' need, when there is a risk for either the mother or her baby. If it is suggested to a woman that caesarean section is advantageous to either herself or more significantly her baby, then not surprisingly she will be glad to have the operation.

Certainly in the present study none of the women delivered by emergency caesarean section who were interviewed questioned the need for the operation, although many wanted more information about the events that had led up to it.

An important indicator of women's reactions to their experience of section is their attitude to future pregnancies. Six months after delivery six (14 per cent) of the women delivered by emergency caesarean section were adamant that they would never have another baby compared with only two (4 per cent) in the group delivered vaginally. In five of the six cases the women stated that this decision was the direct result of their labour and delivery experience, whereas in the control group the decision to limit the family to one child was unrelated. A further 7 (17 per cent) women in the study group were unsure if they would have another baby and in 4 cases again this was a result of their intrapartum experience. Of the 7 (16 per cent) women in the control group who were unsure about a future pregnancy, only one said that this was related to her experience on this occasion, although it was postnatal problems rather than traumatic labour events.

Women delivered by caesarean section took significantly longer than those delivered vaginally to feel close to their infants and these differences persisted for several months after the birth. Only 18 (36 per cent) women in the study group stated that they felt close to the baby immediately compared with 28 (56 per cent) in the control group. By one month after delivery 24 (48 per cent) women in the study group felt close to the baby compared with 38 (76 per cent) in the control group and by two months after the birth there was still a significant statistical difference between the two groups, with 30 (60 per cent) of the study population and 41 (82 per cent) of the controls feeling close to the baby. No statistical difference at any point was found in the control group between those women delivered by forceps and those delivered spontaneously.

Of the 15 women who took longer than two months to feel close to their infant only two did not see the baby at the time of delivery. However, contact with the infant in the 24 hours following delivery appeared to be limited in all cases (usually because of admission to the Special Care Baby Unit) and 12 of the 15 women did not feed the baby until after this time. The promotion of bonding between the mother and her infant has become an increasingly important part of midwifery and obstetric care. Bonding is characterized as being primarily undirectional, occurring rapidly and facilitated by

physical contact (Reading 1983). Several studies have shown that
the hour after birth is a particularly sensitive time and that bonding
between parents and their infants can be enhanced by allowing them
the maximum opportunity to feed, feel and hold their baby (Klaus *et
al.* 1972; Kennel *et al.* 1974; De Chateau 1980).

The performance of an emergency caesarean section will inevitably
influence the amount of contact a mother has with her baby in the
hour after delivery and in addition maternal reactions are likely to
be affected by the stress associated with the operation. In the present
study all of the women had less than ninety minutes to prepare
themselves for the operation and 80 per cent knew of the decision for
less than an hour before going to theatre. When told of the decision
many of the women felt exhausted, frightened, confused or detached.
Although 70 per cent of the group saw the baby immediately at
delivery only 20 per cent actually held the baby in theatre and this
was usually just for a few moments before the infant was taken away.
Almost half of the women did not hold their baby in the 12 hours after
delivery and 76 per cent did not feed the baby in the twenty-four hour
period following the birth. In contrast 90 per cent of the control group
held the baby immediately and 92 per cent had fed the infant within
twenty-four hours. Seventy per cent of the women delivered vaginally
were allowed some time alone with the baby and their partner after
delivery although in over 70 per cent of these cases the duration of
such contact was less than half an hour.

Klaus and Kennel (1982) have suggested that separation of the
mother and infant after delivery may have adverse effects on
maternal attachment which can persist for several months. All
women delivered by caesarean section in the hospital where the
study was carried out are admitted to a Special Care Unit for a
variable period of time following the birth. This unit has no nursery
facilities and babies are kept in the ward nurseries and brought up to
the mothers at feeding time. The purpose of the Special Care Unit is
to provide extra support and rest for women who have experienced
difficult deliveries or other problems after birth. In the study group,
8 (16 per cent) women would have preferred to go directly to a
postnatal ward from theatre, either because they did not like being
separated from the baby or because they were bored in the unit.
At the other end of the spectrum, 18 (36 per cent) felt that they
were not in the unit for long enough and were expected to do far
too much for themselves in the postnatal wards. Overall 26 (52 per
cent) women appreciated admission to the Special Care Unit as they

were tired and sore in the first forty-eight hours after surgery and it allowed them to rest. Seventeen women (34 per cent) would have appreciated more time with the baby during the stay and 6 (12 per cent) said they were unable to rest properly because they were so worried that something was wrong with their infant. Such findings highlight the fact that different individuals have different needs and these must be considered if the most appropriate care is to be given. In the light of these findings, it is probably not surprising that women in the study group took longer than those in the control group to feel close to their infants.

Examination of the comments made by women in both the study and control groups at the time of both the hospital and home interviews revealed deficiencies in some aspects of the care they received. The distinct themes that were apparent were:

1 Lack of realistic preparation for labour, delivery and parenthood;
2 Lack of support and conflicting advice from midwives, especially in the postnatal wards;
3 Failure of communication between women and staff; it was apparent that this occurred in all areas from antenatal care to the postnatal wards.

Each of these areas will be considered in more detail.

Prenatal education

Antenatal preparation classes should play an important role in preparing women for pregnancy, delivery and parenthood and in the present study 76 per cent of women in both the study and control groups attended a class on at least one occasion. Recent research has criticized the content of antenatal classes and questioned the teaching abilities of midwives and health visitors (Murphy-Black and Faulkner 1988). Such criticism includes:

- poor preparation of sessions;
- conflicting advice given;
- lack of realism about the burdens of parenthood;
- giving the wrong impression.

Midwives have little preparation for teaching and Myles's (1985) suggestion that midwives' 'expert knowledge of midwifery and vast experience in dealing with women during pregnancy and labour qualify them as unrivalled teachers of expectant mothers' would appear over-optimistic. A major problem of parent-craft teaching is the didactic style frequently adopted by the teachers. Inevitably antenatal classes will have participants of mixed needs and abilities and good antenatal teaching requires staff to be responsive to the needs of individual women and their partners. This involves allowing the participants to direct the choice of topics to be discussed.

Antenatal classes were criticized by 24 of the women (13 study, 11 control). The women felt that the teaching in these classes did not adequately prepare them for the experience of labour and coping with the new arrival afterwards. Many women expected to cope with the pain of labour by utilizing the breathing exercises and positions taught in the classes and were shocked by the intensity of the pain actually experienced. Women also felt that the classes did not prepare them for any deviations from the course of normal labour such as slow progress or operative delivery. Explanations of caesarean section at classes was limited to elective deliveries for breech presentation and no mention was made of emergency sections during the course of labour.

Women also complained that little attention was paid to the problems that might occur in the postnatal period. Several women said that the parentcraft sisters only stressed the positive aspects of breastfeeding and failed to highlight the difficulties which may arise in establishing this method of feeding. In retrospect some felt that if these potential problems had been discussed beforehand, they might have been better able to cope with difficulties as they arose. Some of the other topics that women felt should have been included in the teaching were postnatal depression (as opposed to third-day 'blues'), support available in the community for mothers with new babies and how to cope with perineal pain and the aftermath of a caesarean section. One woman also mentioned that she had bled intermittently for several weeks after delivery and was terrified 'that her insides were coming out', only to discover at the postnatal visit that this was a relatively common occurrence. A number of women felt that it would be helpful to have discussions on the changes that occur in family relationships and life-style with the arrival of a new baby.

From some of the comments made by the women it would appear that in attempting to instil a positive attitude towards labour and delivery and the achievement of a spontaneous delivery, topics such as forceps delivery and caesarean section were played down or even ignored. As it is impossible to predict all those women who may require caesarean section prior to the onset of labour, it would seem reasonable that some information about caesarean section should be given at these classes. During the year of the study in the hospital where the research was conducted, 16 per cent of primigravidae had caesarean deliveries and a further 28 per cent were delivered by forceps, so almost half had other than 'normal' deliveries. As primigravidae are the main attenders at such classes it would seem appropriate that some discussion of alternative delivery modes should be encouraged.

Postnatal care

The second report of the Maternity Services Advisory Committee (1984) recognized that postnatal care is as important a part of the childbearing process as the actual delivery yet noted that in many units it had the lowest priority. 'Inadequate and under qualified care' resulted in communication failure, conflicting advice, confusion and lack of maternal satisfaction. The report emphasized the importance of meeting both the physical and emotional needs of the mother during this vital time. In the present study postnatal care was the area most frequently criticized and comments were made as often in the control group as the study group. Some of this was directed to the physical environment within the wards, where capital expenditure would be needed to meet criticisms about the lack of appropriate facilities. Other criticisms related to areas where change might be brought about more easily.

One of the most important objectives of postnatal care is to promote the physical recovery of the mother and yet at the time of the hospital interview, 44 per cent of the study group and 24 per cent of the controls felt they didn't get adequate rest or had difficulty in sleeping in hospital. When interviewed at home, 33 per cent of the women reiterated this problem and felt that something should be done to improve this aspect of postnatal care. Many of the wards in the hospital are open-plan or of a 'Nightingale' design and inevitably when babies are kept beside their mothers the problem of noise arises. However, in many cases women complained that the sleeping difficulties were caused by staff conversations, or televisions or lights being left on; sensitivity on the part of the staff might have minimized these problems.

Over 25 per cent of the women interviewed (15 study, 7 control) were critical of the support given to them by the midwives in the postnatal wards. Many of these women spoke of feeling abandoned in the wards and left to get on with things without assistance:

> I felt they expected you to do far too much in the postnatal wards. Although it was busy they just left you most of the time. There was lots I wanted to ask and I ended up weeping for most of the time.

Another woman found the obstetric students on secondment from general training to be the most helpful. All of the women delivered by caesarean section who made comments on postnatal care said they felt the midwives were unaware of the difficulties they had both physically and psychologically, in coping with the 'aftermath' of this method of delivery:

> The midwives forgot how the baby had been delivered and when I developed a temperature nobody seemed to bother – that wouldn't happen in a surgical ward.

and

> I felt the staff weren't very sympathetic to how I felt about my labour. One of the midwives was quite sharp and told me I should think myself lucky that I had a healthy baby. I seemed to spend most of the time weeping.

Sixty-eight per cent of the study group said they found it difficult to cope with the physical care of the baby at the time of the hospital interview. These difficulties were related to lifting and handling the baby, getting in and out of bed, bending and finding a comfortable position in which to feed the baby. Several of the women felt that it would be helpful to have a ward set aside for those delivered by caesarean section which was equipped with either beds with adjustable height control or stools to help the women get in and out of bed. Some also felt that the mutual support that would be afforded by this arrangement would be beneficial. A further advantage of this kind of ward would be that the midwifery staff would be more aware that these women might need more help with the physical aspects of baby care. Interestingly a number of women in the control group mentioned that they had had to help women delivered by section in the wards, because there were too few staff to attend to their needs.

It was apparent from interviewing women in the caesarean group, especially those delivered under general anaesthesia, that the sequence of events leading up to the decision to operate and immediately prior to the operation was often confused. All of the women delivered under general anaesthesia mentioned that they

had difficulty recalling events immediately following delivery. The
length of time that was 'blurred' or 'missing' ranged from a day to
several days. Typical comments made by the women included

> The next couple of days are a blur too, I just remember sleeping
> and wakening. Now people have told me things that happened but
> I can't remember them.

and

> The next 2–3 days are completely blank, apparently I didn't
> even want to see the baby. They took me up to the paediatric
> department but I hardly remember being there.

Two of the women said they had difficulty assimilating the fact that
they had a baby during this time:

> When they brought me the baby I thought she was my sister when
> she was a baby. I found it difficult to believe she was mine.

One woman was very unhappy with the information given by the
staff and said,

> When I asked the nurse what I'd had she just walked away – I
> had to phone home and reverse the charges to get details.

Clarifying the confusion and allowing the women the opportunity
to reconstruct their experiences and express their feelings is an
important and often neglected part of facilitating adjustment in
the postnatal period. Midwives have an important role to play in
counselling in this area.

Conflicting advice from midwives was identified by many women
and this was usually related to the area of infant feeding. A number
of women were still angry at the time of the home interview about
the care they received in this area. Many of the women felt that their
confidence was undermined by the conflicting professional advice
given and ultimately this resulted in a number of them giving up
breastfeeding.

Klaus and Kennel (1982) maintain that certain influences which
affect mother–child relationships are fixed, whilst others such as
hospital practices and the attitudes of staff are alterable and may
be changed to improve the establishment of maternal relationships.
Ball (1987) found that the delivery of midwifery care had an effect on
the transition to motherhood and could, by increasing or decreasing
stress in mothers, make a notable difference to the way she adapted

to the demands of mothering the child. Some of the factors which were shown to affect stress levels were conflicting advice from midwives, which reduced the mother's self-image in feeding; rest; lack of continuity of information between midwives and the fact that most postnatal care seemed to be planned on a routinized basis with a chronological succession of increasing responsibility for the care of the infant by the mother, irrespective of her age, condition after delivery or previous childbearing experiences.

Postnatal-care which is planned on a routinized system is insufficiently flexible and sensitive to allow the best possible support of the mother. Increasingly midwives have recognized that such systems need to be replaced with evaluated individualized care based on the available information. The midwifery and nursing process is a systematic problem-solving or problem-preventing approach to care which involves an acceptance of the woman's right to individualized care and to active participation in that care, including decision making (Ashworth 1981). It is used to assess individual needs, plan and deliver appropriate care to meet the identified needs; finally the effect of the care is evaluated. The process is ongoing and should be used from the booking visit until discharge by the community midwives after delivery. The single record ensures that all those involved in the delivery of care know what has been decided, thus ensuring continuity.

The midwifery process was adopted in the hospital where the research was conducted in 1981 and had been in operation for a number of years when the present study commenced. The areas of postnatal care found to be deficient in the present study are the same areas frequently cited in other studies, so it was particularly disappointing to find that routine, mechanistic care is still apparently being given.

Communication

Failure of communication is the most frequently complained of aspect of maternity care. Although this can occur in other medical and surgical fields, it appears that resentment about, or criticism of, poor communications is more acute in the maternity service than in any other area (MacIntyre 1982). Several studies have shown that women are often dissatisfied with the lack of opportunities made available to them to ask questions and the quality of the information and explanations given to them by care-givers. This may occur in the course of antenatal care (Reid and McIlwaine 1980; MacIntyre 1982), in the intrapartum period (Kirke 1980; Kirkham 1981) or in the postnatal period (Ball 1987).

Failures of communication were seen on a number of occasions in the present study and occurred in both women delivered vaginally and by caesarean section.

Some women mentioned the support given to them in the labour ward by both the midwives and obstetricians. In the control group, of the 28 women who made some comment about the labour ward staff, only 3 felt that the midwives could have been more supportive. In the study group, 32 women commented on the support given by staff and generally the comments were of a less positive nature. Twelve women were happy with the midwives and doctors but a further 7 felt they should have been given more information about what was happening or that the staff could have been more sympathetic towards them:

The staff were very helpful but I would have appreciated more information about how my labour was coming on.

I felt the midwives were very supportive but I feel quite angry about the attitude of the doctors who were very secretive about what was happening.

I was annoyed with the registrar who wanted the epidural to wear off so that I could push. He wasn't at all sympathetic, I couldn't cope with the pain and had to beg for them to top it up.

Some of the women commented on the fact that although explanations may have been given by the staff, events happened too quickly and they were unable to take in information. Typical comments made by these women included

The staff were very supportive but with so much happening I didn't really take much in.

The support was good from the midwives and they explained what was happening, but ultimately it didn't resolve what I was feeling [disappointment, confusion, or bewilderment].

The baby's heart was going off and I remember being pushed from side to side and then put on a trolley. I can't remember if anyone told me what was going to happen, it was all such a rush and I just wanted it over.

A further 12 women were unhappy with the support given by the staff during labour; the reasons for this ranged from procedures which were carried out without consent:

> They kept on giving me injections to stop it [nausea], which didn't work and I didn't really want them, however they never really asked me;

not believing the women:

> They didn't give me any information and wouldn't admit to the fact that I was in labour;

to not allowing the women to participate in the decision-making process:

> I didn't feel involved in decisions that were made about me.

It is of concern to note that three months after delivery, 20 per cent of women in the study group either did not know why the caesarean section was carried out or gave completely mistaken explanations for the performance of the operation. A further 16 per cent were only partially right in their comprehension. It may have been that these women were given the reasons for it at a time when they were unable to take in fully what was said or that the explanations were given in a way that they were unable to understand. There may also have been confusion among the medical and midwifery staff or an assumption that the reasons had already been given by someone else. Some of the women interviewed said that they had never been told directly what had occurred but had gleaned information from overheard conversations between doctors or doctors and midwives.

At the time of the home interview it was apparent that 8 (19 per cent) of the 42 women delivered by caesarean section who were interviewed had little or no information about the events which occurred in labour and resulted in operative delivery and had implications for the management of future pregnancies. One woman complained that no one had told her personally how her next baby would be delivered but that she had overheard the consultant say to a registrar that as it was a failed forceps delivery she would have an elective section next time.

Irrespective of why communication failures arose, it is apparent from these findings that provision must be made to allow the woman to discuss the events of labour and the reasons for any operative intervention. To ensure that no cases are overlooked it should be recorded in both the obstetric and midwifery notes. Discussion should also include the likely management of future pregnancies. The ideal timing of such discussion will depend on the woman's individual situation, but given that some women did not attend the postnatal examination and others are likely to attend the general practitioner rather than the hospital, the responsibility should lie with the hospital staff to ensure that it takes place before hospital discharge.

Auditing for change

The results of the present study emphasize the need for staff involved in maternity care to undertake systematic evaluation of the care given throughout the antenatal, intrapartum and postnatal period. Inherent within the Code of Professional Conduct of the UK Central Council for Nursing, Midwifery and Health Visiting is the concept of accountability for professional practice. Midwives are responsible for planning, delivering and *evaluating* any care given in the course of practice. The importance of evaluation and quality assurance in nursing and midwifery practice is emphasized in the two recent strategy documents published by the Department of Health (1989) and the Scottish Home and Health Department (1990). One of the key objectives in the latter document is, 'to ensure that standards of [nursing] care are developed and monitored, and a system for Nursing Audit is established'.

However, professional practice must also be responsive to the needs of the consumer, and therefore audit must also take into account the views and opinions of clients patients. These views on the quality of the health service are increasingly being sought by both managers and health care professionals. Nurses and midwives usually work as part of a multi-disciplinary team, but because of the close relationships they often form with those using the health care system, have a key role to play in the overall evaluation of the delivery of care. All midwives who are actively and directly engaged in professional practice must ensure that these goals are promoted and achieved.

References

Affonso, D. and Stichler, J. (1980) 'Cesarean birth: Women's reactions', *American Journal of Nursing* March: 468–70.

Ashworth, P. (1981) 'The midwifery/nursing process at home and abroad', in proceedings from the conference 'Research and the midwife', November 1981, Dept. of Nursing Studies, University of Manchester: 2–15.

Ball, J. A. (1987) *Reactions to Motherhood: The Role of Postnatal Care*, Cambridge:

Cambridge University Press.
Boyd, C., Francome, C., Bartley, D., Evans, R. (1983) *One Birth in Nine: Caesarean Section Trends Since 1978*, London: The Maternity Alliance.
Chalmers, I. (1980) 'An introduction to perinatal audit and surveillance', in I. Chalmers and G. McIlwaine (eds) *Perinatal Audit and Surveillance*, London: Royal College of Obstetrician, and Gynaecologists.
Cranley, M. S., Hedahl, K. J., Pegg, S. (1983) 'Women's perceptions of vaginal and cesarean deliveries', *Nursing Research* 32: 10–15.
De Chateau, P. (1980) 'The first hour after delivery – its impact on the synchrony of the parent–infant relationship', *Paediatrician* 9: 151–68.
Department of Health (1989) *A Strategy for Nursing*, London: Department of Health.
Erb, L., Hill, G., Houston, D. (1983) 'A survey of parents' attitudes toward their cesarean births in Manitoba hospitals', *Birth* 10: 85–91.
Her Majesty's Stationery Office (1989) *Working for Patients* Cm. 555, London: HMSO.
Information and Statistics Division (1989) *Hospital and Health Board Comparisons in Obstetrics: 1985-1987*, Edinburgh: Common Services Agency.
Janis, I. L. (1958) *Psychological Stress: Psychoanalytic and Behavioral Studies of Surgical Patients*, New York: John Wiley.
Kennel, J. H., Jerauld, R., Wolfe, H. *et al.* (1974) 'Maternal behaviour one year after early and extended postpartum contact', *Developmental Medicine and Child Neurology* 16: 172–9.
Kirke, P. N. (1980) 'Mothers' views of obstetric care', *British Journal of Obstetrics and Gynaecology* 87: 1029–33.
Kirkham, M. (1981) 'Information giving by midwives during labour', in proceedings from the conference 'Research and the midwife', November 1981, Dept. of Nursing Studies, University of Manchester: 38–50.
Klaus, M. H. and Kennel, J. H. (1982) *Parent Infant Bonding*, St Louis, Mo.: Mosby.
Klaus, M. H., Jerauld, R., Kreger, B., McAlpine, W., Steffa, M., Kennel, J. H. (1972) 'Maternal attachment: Importance of the first postpartum days', *New England Journal of Medicine* 286: 460–3.
McIlwaine, G. M., Cole, S. K., Macnaughton, M. C. (1985) 'The rising caesarean section rate – a matter of concern?', *Health Bulletin* 43: 301–5.
MacIntyre, S. (1982) 'Communications between pregnant women and their medical and midwifery attendants', *Midwives' Chronicle and Nursing Notes* 95: 387–94.
Marut, J. S., Mercer, R. T. (1979) 'Comparison of primiparas' perceptions of vaginal and cesarean births', *Nursing Research* 28: 260–6.
Maternity Services Advisory Committee (1984) *Maternity Care in Action, Part II: Care During Childbirth*, London: HMSO.
Murphy-Black, T. and Faulkner, A. (1988) *Antenatal Group Skills Training*, Edinburgh: John Wiley.
Myles, M. (1985) *Textbook for Midwives, 10th edn.*, Edinburgh: Churchill Livingstone.
Oakley, A. (1980) *Women Confined*, Oxford: Martin Robertson.
Oakley, A. (1983) 'Social consequences of obstetric technology: The importance of measuring "soft" outcomes', *Birth* 10: 99–108.

O'Driscoll, K., Foley, M. (1983) 'Correlation of decrease in perinatal mortality and increase in cesarean section rates', *Obstetrics and Gynecology* 61: 1–5.

Pearson, J. W. (1984) 'Cesarean section and perinatal mortality', *American Journal of Obstetrics and Gynecology* 148: 155–9.

Placek, P. J., Taffel, S. M. (1980) 'Trends in cesarean section rates for the United States 1970–78', *Public Health Reports* 95: 540–8.

Placek, P. J., Taffel, S. M., Moien, M. S. (1988) '1986 c-sections rise: VBAC's inch upward', *American Journal of Public Health* 7: 562–3.

Raines, E. (1984) 'Professional liability in perspective', *Obstetrics and Gynecology* 63: 839–45.

Reading, A. J. (1983) 'Bonding', in J. Studd (ed.) *Progress in Obstetrics and Gynaecology*, Vol. III, Edinburgh: Churchill Livingstone, 128–36.

Reid, M., McIlwaine, G. (1980) 'Consumer opinion of a hospital antenatal clinic', *Social Science and Medicine* 14a: 363–8.

Rosen, M. G. (1981) *Cesarean Childbirth: Report of a Consensus Development Conference* (NIH Publication no. 82–2067), Bethesda, Md.: National Institute of Health.

Scottish Home and Health Department (1990) *A Strategy for Nursing, Midwifery and Health Visiting in Scotland*, Edinburgh: HMSO.

Shearer, M. H. (1983) 'The difficulty of measuring satisfaction with perinatal care', *Birth* 10: 77.

Thiery, M. and Derom, R. (1986a) 'Review of evaluative studies on caesarean section, Part I: Trends in caesarean section and perinatal mortality', in M. Kaminiski, B. Gerard, P. Buekins, H. J. Huisjes, G. McIlwaine, H. K. Selbman (eds) *Perinatal Care Delivery Systems*, Oxford: Oxford University Press: 93–113.

Thiery, M. and Derom, R. (1986b) 'Review of evaluative studies on caesarean section, Part II: Specific obstetric problems related to increasing caesarean section rates and risks of caesarean section', in M. Kaminiski, B. Gerard, P. Buekins, H. J., Huisjes, G. McIlwaine, H. K. Selbman (eds) *Perinatal Care Delivery Systems*, Oxford: Oxford University Press: 129–55.

Chapter 10

Answering back
The role of respondents in women's health research

Helen Roberts

Well quite honestly, I said, I hope this research is worth it. I said to my mum, I've got this lady coming to see me this morning. She said, 'What about?' I said, I hope it's not a load of old rubbish. Because there's been so much research on such rubbishy things I feel money's been wasted. So she said, 'Oh it probably is . . .' Well, it's a bit indulgent isn't it, really, just talking about yourself all the time?

(Oakley 1979: 309)

I would just like to thank everyone involved in this questionnaire because it has made me realise a lot of my feelings and help do something about them.

(Questionnaire 2: 0610, Pritchard and Teo, forthcoming)

From randomized clinical trials to the 'softest' of social research on women's health, the respondent, participant, or 'subject' of the research is crucial to the enterprise. Research on women's health cannot be carried out without women participating, knowingly or not, in the research process. They may be relatively passive participants, taking a particular drug, or having a particular procedure carried out, with the results simply being observed; there may be no real part played by the main players, the patients, other than taking the drugs and recovering or not. Or they may have their opinions actively sought about the desirability of a particular service such as family planning or well women's clinics; they may be questioned on their willingness or otherwise to participate in breast or cervical screening or they may be asked to describe their experience of maternity care. In the finished research 'product', however, the respondents are normally curiously absent. The absence of the respondents from many finished research projects is indicative of their objectification throughout the research. They are there right up until the last moment, and then they are excluded. They are made mere objects from the beginning, and the human material for the research is frequently relegated to the position of inhabitants of a different world from that of the observer.

In reports of clinical trials or case reports in the medical literature for instance, doctors referring patients to a particular trial, or drawing a colleague's attention to an 'interesting case', are frequently acknowledged while the patients themselves may go entirely unacknowledged. An issue of the *British Journal of Obstetrics and Gynaecology* (1990), chosen at random, contained a mix of case-studies, trials and other studies, as well as commentaries and research reports. Some of the articles described studies which required no active co-operation from women. Their tissue was examined, or they were entered into a study, and the outcome reported required no conscious input from the women. Other studies required varying degrees of time, effort or discomfort. (One, which required thirty-six women to agree to an extra venesection at delivery, is confusingly entitled 'Determinants of fetal and maternal atrial natiuretic peptide concentrations at delivery *in man*' (my emphasis) (Voto *et al*. 1990: 1123).) As well as blood tests, women who provided the raw data for the articles in this journal also provided urine, tissue, diary cards and symptom questionnaires (in one case completed on 7 occasions by a set of respondents). Table 10.1 shows the pattern of acknowledgements in the fourteen articles which comprised this issue of the journal.

Table 10.1 Acknowledgements appearing in obstetrics and gynaecology journal

Acknowledgements to:	
No one	3
Funders	8
Colleagues	5
Clinic staff	1
Computing help	1
Preparation of the manuscript	4
Total no. of articles:	14

While no paper acknowledged the patients, one acknowledged

the assistance of a nurse in 'the management of patients' and others acknowledged colleagues for 'access to the clinical records of patients under their care'. That it is possible to extend the courtesy of acknowledgement to the women who participate in research in a scientific article may be seen in the acknowledgements to the scholarly report on the Canadian multi-centre trial of chorion villus sampling and amniocentesis; in it the participants are thanked before the funders: 'We thank the women who, generously and altruistically, took part in this study . . .' (Canadian collaborative CVS-amniocentesis clinical trial group 1989: 6)

Frankly acknowledging and drawing on the special part played in research by respondents in the way which Ann Oakley did in her study *Becoming a Mother* quoted above is rare. This chapter looks at some of the literature on the role of research respondents, discusses in a preliminary way the costs and benefits to respondents of participation in research, and describes a number of ethical issues involved in the participation of live human subjects in research. Finally, using as an example the final page of a questionnaire of a Scottish study, 'Women's experiences during pregnancy', which is being conducted by Colin Pritchard and Philip Teo, this chapter looks at respondents' views as a largely untapped area of expertise on women's health.

In some large-scale studies, research respondents may be at several removes from a piece of research, particularly where secondary analyses are concerned. The General Household Survey (GHS) for instance, on which some of the data in Jennie Popay's chapter are based, collects data from a very large number of households, and respondents are, of course, aware that this is part of a research enterprise. The detailed analyses of GHS data to look at, for instance, sex differences in sickness absence and care of the elderly (Arber 1990) or differences in health and health status between men and women may not have been foreseen by the original research respondents, but it is difficult to foresee any undesirable consequences for those who participated in the survey. This is not always the case. In some clinical research, women may not always be aware that as well as receiving treatment, they are also the subjects of research. A patient who found herself in two randomized clinical trials without her knowledge or consent subsequently wrote, 'Withholding information about the trials may have invalidated them. It was forgotten that patients, unlike laboratory animals, can move around and communicate with each other. Treatments are discussed and unexplained differences discovered . . . the stress produced may be the very factors which affect health and well being' (Thomas 1988). Meanwhile, some doctors argue that it is wrong to inform patients with life-threatening illnesses that one treatment or another means that they are entered into one arm or another of a clinical trial, since this may be an added source of stress: 'If protection of the subject is the reason for obtaining informed consent, the possibility of iatrogenic harm to the subject as a direct result of the consent ritual must be considered' (Loftus and Fries 1979: 11). As Ann Oakley points out, the term 'ritual', used in a derogatory sense, gives a view of how these investigators regard the task of informing people what is being done to them (Oakley 1990). The research design described in this collection by Rona McCandlish and Mary Renfrew is, of course, at the extreme other end of the spectrum of information and consent, which brings its own problems.

Research published in 1990 in *The Lancet* compared the survival of a group of women with breast cancer undergoing only conventional treatment with a group who supplemented conventional treatment with the more holistic therapies of the Bristol Cancer Help Centre (Bagenal *et al.* 1990). Early results, which were the subject of a press conference and therefore attracted wide publicity outside the medical press, indicated a reduced survival period in the group who had attended the Bristol Cancer Help Centre. Within a few weeks, attention had been drawn to a number of serious methodological flaws in the study (Hayes *et al.* 1990; Heyse-Moor 1990; Munro and Payne 1990). The director of research of one the funding organizations involved wrote, 'Our own evaluation is that the study's results can be explained by the fact that women going to Bristol had more severe disease than control women' (Bodmer 1990: 1188).

Less prominence was given in the national press to criticisms of the study. While many research subjects are not in a position to be aware of, let alone comment on, research to which they have contributed, the wide publicity given to this study meant that few of the women who had participated could have been unaware of the initial findings. Thus, late entries to the public debate over this study were some of the research subjects themselves. In a letter to a national newspaper, one wrote, 'As one of the women surveyed in the ill-fated *Lancet* study, I . . . am at a turning point. Serious issues arise for patients who are used in such surveys. A support group is being formed to share experiences and to consider what action should be taken' (Goodare 1990: 16).

The role of research respondents in women's health research

Those who are researched, as others have noted, are more likely to be the powerless than the powerful: patients are more likely to come under scrutiny than hospital consultants or general managers in the National Health Service and are less likely to have the opportunity to comment on such scrutiny.

A great deal of research on health depends on the good will, participation and time of women, although the choice of women as respondents is not always dictated by an overwhelming desire to explore women's needs and experiences as such. Women may become research respondents because they are less willing to slam the door on the researcher, more likely than are men to be socialized to want to be helpful, and because they are perceived as being more flexible in relation to demands on their time, a misconception discussed in Jennie Popay's chapter in this collection.

George Brown and Tirril Harris, whose work on depression among women is a classic, frankly admitted,

> We needed as many people as possible to agree to co-operate in what we knew would be a lengthy interview. Such an interviewing programme is expensive and one way to reduce its cost was to study women only, as they probably suffer from depression more than men. It also seemed likely that women, who are more often at home during the day, would be more willing to agree to see us for several hours.
>
> (Brown and Harris 1978: 22)

Women's willingness to act as respondents is a compelling reason to use them as such. The time after the birth of a child is unlikely to be the most leisured period in a woman's life, yet surveys conducted to explore women's experiences of childbirth can expect responses of at least 75 per cent (Mason 1989: 1) which compares very favourably with responses to research enquiries from medical practitioners.

Given the importance of human subjects to research on health, it is perhaps surprising that the role of women as participants in research has received little more attention than the role of the rats in the physiology department animal house (and perhaps rather less, since the interest taken in the latter by the Animal Liberation Front). With the exception of Hilary Graham's (1983, 1984) work, such literature as there is tends to concentrate on ethical matters. The questions of whether researchers are doing right by their respondents; whether they are benefiting or harming them; whether respondents are active participants in research or unwitting 'subjects', are important and deserve the serious attention they have received. Marina Barnard's chapter in this collection represents a contribution to this genre. From a feminist perspective, Ann Oakley's article on interviewing women (Oakley 1981) and Janet Finch's discussion of the ethics and politics of interviewing women (Finch 1984) are classics.

Other aspects of the role of respondents have been less thoroughly explored. In an early research project in which I was involved, looking at variations in consultation rates in middle-aged women at the general practitioner's surgery (Roberts 1981), I became uncomfortably aware that research respondents may have an agenda of their own, quite at variance with that which interests the researcher. Just as a doctor taking a history may discard those symptoms which seem important to the patient, but which don't fit a particular 'story' or disease pattern, so researchers may prefer to frame their questions so as to induce the minimum of 'interference' from respondents. It is clearly simpler, more convenient, and will lead to less equivocal research results to ask a woman to rate the discomfort from her episiotomy on a scale of 1 to 5 than to ask her a more general question about her experience of childbirth. General or so-called 'open' questions may be difficult for respondents to answer, are untidy and time-consuming at the analysis stage, and at the end of the day may be difficult to use. There is an understandable tendency in research reports where responses to open questions are used, to concentrate examples on those women providing witty, unusual or otherwise colourful responses. Val Mason, whose survey manual provides an excellent guide to those wishing to carry out a survey into women's experiences of maternity care, suggests:

[Open questions] are less likely to be answered fully, for example by groups such as those with no educational qualifications and those for whom English is not their first language. . . . [Responses] can provide useful illustrative material in a survey report. Indeed they can bring to life for the reader the experiences behind the necessarily more standardised answers printed in the questionnaire.

(Mason 1989: 17)

Respondents' voices

As an example of the sorts of things respondents may contribute to a study when given a free rein, I refer below to one aspect of a Glasgow study currently in progress exploring women's experiences during pregnancy (Pritchard and Teo, forthcoming). The study is designed to assess the stressfulness of daily social roles. The emphasis is on the persistent and continuing problems and difficulties encountered by pregnant women in the course of their daily lives and the extent to which these are translated into the experience of stress. The study consists of two antenatal self-completed questionnaires at 20 and 30 weeks gestation and data on the course, management and outcome of pregnancy from case-note abstraction. In common with other well-planned surveys, the response rate to this one has been high (in excess of 70 per cent), and a formidable range of data have been collected and are in the process of analysis. The questionnaires were well designed, easing the respondent through a fairly lengthy series of questions, helping her to bypass those questions irrelevant to her situation and providing appropriate guidance to secure optimal response. As one respondent wrote,

> I'm very pleased with the lay-out of this booklet . . . and I think if it can help others, well good enough.
>
> (Questionnaire 1: 0054)

The A4-sized questionnaire was put together in a booklet format, a design which apparently had some bearing on the way in which it was perceived by respondents. Booklets received during pregnancy tend to be aimed at providing something: information, advice or help of some kind, and a number of respondents clearly viewed the questionnaire in this light:

> Having books like this makes me feel confident about my pregnancy to know that there is research being done to help people through pregnancy.
>
> (Questionnaire 1: 0052)

> I think this booklet is very good as it can help a lot of people. It's a very good idea. And thank you for giving me the chance to let you know how I feel as it's very hard for me this time.
>
> (Questionnaire 1: 0060)

The results of this study will be reported elsewhere (Pritchard and Teo forthcoming), and the aspect which I discuss below relates to only one page of two lengthy questionnaires. At the end of each questionnaire, an A4-sized page was left blank, apart from the following invitation:

> Now that you have answered all our questions, it would help us if you have any comments that you would like to make. We would be specially interested if you have anything to say about this booklet or about your pregnancy and the care you are getting. Please use the space below to write anything you want to say.

Although an invitation to respondents to comment on research is not unique, it is not standard practice. It is, however, good practice, and the invitation above allowed respondents to comment both on the questionnaire and on areas of their pregnancy or their care which were not addressed in the questions asked. It is perhaps testimony to women's desire to contribute to research in this area that over half the respondents took the opportunity to comment. It should be remembered that the women doing so were in the last few months of pregnancy, all had another child to care for, some were in addition in paid employment and all had domestic responsibilities. It was clear from handwriting and spelling (for which women frequently and needlessly apologized) that the comments were by no means restricted to women who had had the benefit of further and higher education.

> I hope I have been able to help you with your questionnaire. I am sorry for any mistakes I have made and hope you understand my answers.
>
> (Questionnaire 1: 228)

As in Oakley's (1979) work and other studies, the comments revealed a desire to help other women in the same situation as an important motivation in completing the questionnaire:

> I . . . like to take part in research work. I think it's good that people take an interest in research work specially about pregnant people.
>
> (Questionnaire 2: 441)

The extent to which respondents, who had donated their time to the research, thanked the researchers for 'listening' was striking, and has been remarked upon in other studies (Oakley, McPherson and Roberts 1990).

Thank you for letting me help you.

(Questionnaire 2: 0060)

Ann Oakley's chapter in this collection refers to the therapeutic potential of research, and a number of respondents to this study tend to confirm her view:

The booklet is very good as it makes you sit down and think about yourself for a change. As I usually spend so much of my time thinking about other people's problems I am apt to have no time to think of my own like the fact I do get depressed but try not to show it or even admit it to myself.

(Questionnaire 2: 0563)

I like the booklet very much. You can tell someone your problems without facing them.

(Questionnaire 2: 0352)

I feel this booklet has helped me cope with my pregnancy. It's good to know you are not the only one who is feeling down and unwell.

(Questionnaire 1: 0637)

One respondent described in some detail her physical and emotional problems during the pregnancy and wrote,

I would be interested in your opinion about my feelings put down in this booklet. Anything that helps women during pregnancy has got to be worthwhile . . . . I really appreciate getting the chance to tell someone about this. I only hope you find some use for the information.

(Questionnaire 1: 201)

She was not the only respondent who was concerned about the outcome of the study. One respondent asked,

Why do you want to know all this for? and what will the outcome be? I know it's to improve the health care system, but it's not that you have to improve. It's the waiting to be seen.

(Questionnaire 1: 9476)

Women had helpful comments to make on both the design of the research, and factors which they felt might influence the findings. In this respect, respondents were conscientious in their concern to draw the researchers' attention to what they felt might be problems in interpreting their replies. A particular concern which a number of women pointed out was that strains and stresses varied from day to day. One woman was sent the second questionnaire twice, as her first response was lost in the post. She was good enough to complete it again and wrote,

> I have already completed and returned to you this questionnaire – must have got lost in Christmas post. I think that I have answered some questions differently since a few weeks ago, but this is mainly due to the fact that I am no longer working and therefore have more free time.
>
> (Questionnaire 2: 0446)

Respondents also drew the researchers' attention to the fact that the questions might have been answered very differently in a first pregnancy. In fact both these points had been addressed in the design of the research. Women who already had a child had been chosen in order to avoid as far as possible the confounding effect of marriage and the transition to motherhood in first pregnancies. The questionnaires were administered at 20 and 30 weeks in order to explore differences in response, though some women were clearly puzzled by the similarities in questions asked on the two occasions.

A concern which neatly encapsulates some of the issues which Hilary Graham discusses in her essay 'Do her answers fit his questions? Women and the survey method' (Graham 1983) was raised by one respondent:

> I frequently felt that the answers I gave were not a true reflection of my attitude because the questions themselves did not fit my experience. . . . Not enough attention is paid to the psychological problems a woman, especially a working woman, can face.
>
> (Questionnaire 1: 0354)

She added, in a letter which expanded on some of her concerns,

> I hope your studies lead to at least a degree of improvement in professional attitudes to the psychological problems of pregnancy.

This concern is central to taking seriously the concerns of our respondents, which may sometimes be rather different from our own. Some of the concerns raised by mothers in the Scottish study were frankly practical. Why were waiting times so long at the hospital? Why could that waiting time not be used to better effect? Why was there no crèche? As one mother wrote,

This pregnancy is much more difficult in terms of tiredness and physical problems dealing with another small child e.g. picking them up, going upstairs, unable to get a sleep during the day. I think 2nd time mothers need more help and support, but I think the assumption is that if you've had one normal pregnancy, you should be able to cope without help with the second.

(Questionnaire 2: 0341)

Another referred to the view that second pregnancies are less problematic than first:

I think when you are having your first baby, it is worrying but when it is your second baby, it is more worrying because you know what to expect . . . and you get a little more scared.

(Questionnaire 2: 0380)

There were some direct references by respondents to problems they perceived with the research design. One referred to a question on income:

I think the booklet doesn't go deeply enough to get a true reading. Like the money situation, do you mean our partner's money? or what we are given from our partners? My partner earns high wages but he pays the bills and only gives me money for food . . . I hope this will be of help.

(Questionnaire 2: 168)

There was a feeling that some questions were not sufficiently fine grain to reflect the complexity of people's experience (a problem of which the researchers, were, of course, aware):

I hated the questions where you have a choice of agree, disagree etc. I find them a bit limited and always have to read them a few times to make sure I've understood them the way they were meant.

(Questionnaire 1: 155)

In quite a few instances, it has been very difficult to match an appropriate answer with my response.

(Questionnaire 1: 222)

Some respondents were concerned on the other hand about bias as a result of the length or complexity of the questionnaire:

The questionnaire takes quite a lot of thought to fill in and can be off-putting, hence the time it has taken me to get round to filling it in. I think this will make [it] very selective in who bothers to fill it in – wouldn't it be better to come to the clinic and make use of the time mothers have to sit around. People much prefer talking!

(Questionnaire 1: 0341)

There were a number of ways in which the respondents in the Scottish study used their experience to address research needs. The first and most straightforward way was in responding to the questions framed by the researchers within the terms set for the research. The high response rate and the conscientious way in which respondents drew attention to difficulties indicates the willingness of respondents to take research seriously. The respondents were also taken seriously by the researchers. As one perceptively commented,

About the booklet. I feel you are really grateful for the fact that I have filled in the questions.

and added,

I would like to know really what you are doing with all the information you are gathering.

(Questionnaire 2: 9614)

Occasionally, a respondent would use the comments page to make suggestions about future research. Two women commented on their extraordinarily vivid dreams during pregnancy, and felt that more should be known about this. One had a very specific piece of data which she had brought to the attention of the hospital in the hope that it might help other mothers. Hypothesis formation is not, after all, confined to 'experts':

[During my first pregnancy] my epileptic condition got better and better until the attacks were practically nil. After he was born, I could almost feel some foreign body re-entering and the attacks began again. But although I requested a doctor from the neurological department, no one was informed. Surely if someone had come either myself or someone with the same problem may have benefited . . . If the case is the same this time, I hope someone is informed.

(Questionnaire 1: 9566)

The problem is, how can these experiences be used by researchers in any kind of meaningful way? Mason (1989) suggests a number of alternatives for dealing with the responses to 'open' questions. It might be disappointing to respondents to know that the first option suggested is to carry out no analysis. The second is to simply note whether or not there was a response to the open question, as was done earlier in this chapter. The third option is to list some or all of the open answers with a view to giving the researcher an idea of the range of answers, providing illustrative material for the survey report, and providing the raw material to help develop a coding frame. Such a coding frame involves assigning each answer to a category or a number of categories in order to show the percentages of women giving each category of answer. These are one way forward, but are there other ways in which the richness and diversity of 'free-range' (as opposed to 'battery') data from research respondents might be used?

In practical terms, the needs of funders, researchers and respondents are unlikely to coincide at every point. In the Scottish study quoted above for instance, the researchers' stated (and worthwhile) objective to provide a descriptive 'epidemiology' of psycho-social stress in pregnancy is unlikely to meet the desire of respondents for crèche facilities at the hospital. It may, however, lead indirectly to the improvement in treatment of some of the emotional and psychological consequences of pregnancy which some of the respondents feel is necessary.

It seems to me that there are a number of positive ways in which respondents' views could be used over and above the cosmetic use of apt quotations to enliven research reports. As well as using open comments in the analysis and discussion of a study where appropriate as a matter of course, funding for the following needs to be built into projects:

1 Respondents should receive reports on the findings of the research to which they have contributed, with an invitation to comment.
2 Where hospitals or clinics are used to recruit respondents, they should be sent not only the formal research report, but also any comments made, positive or otherwise, on service provision.
3 Where respondents make recommendations for future research, these should be brought to the attention of funders by way of an appendix.
4 There should be effective dissemination of project findings not simply to academic but also to service providers and wider audiences.

As researchers, we do have particular skills in the collection, analysis and dissemination of research findings (see for example Roberts 1984) but ordinary people use the skills of observation and experience in their everyday lives to make sense of the world in a way which may not be dignified by the lofty term research, but could have similar results. Oakley points out that

> Experience does alter the way people (experts and others) behave: this is part of the scientific method that theories should be tested empirically, not just once under artificial conditions, but constantly in the real world. . . . It is *from* their own experience in this world that most people (who are not scientists) develop their theories, build up their generalisations, become confident about asserting things generally to be true.
>
> (Oakley 1979: 308)

The *intention* of the current imperative to conduct research into 'consumer satisfaction' is unlikely to be targeted towards the use of these kind of data, however freely given they may be, and however cost effective. But in developing health services truly responsive to patients, clients, customers or consumers, we need to take their views seriously, use them effectively, and draw from and build on their knowledge.

The typical concern of social scientists has been with the unique character of research into human subjects which arises from the humanity of the scholar, from the fact that she is both an observer and a part of the thing being observed. But there is another side. For whilst the scholar is also potentially a subject, the subject is potentially as much a source of interpretation, understanding and criticism as is the observer. In their concern to understand the place of their own feelings and suppositions in the interpretation of the human subjects from which they are only artificially, by the process of scholarship, separated, social scientists have been led to neglect the isolation of the thinking object of their research. If the common humanity of object and subject make it impossible for the social scientist to be treated as simply objective, it makes it to the same extent impossible for respondents in a survey to be treated simply as data or the source of data.

What can be learnt from the responses to the survey quoted above? Some of the answers are self-evident, and are provided by the respondents. These also show that the human material of the social scientist is constantly escaping from or simply ignoring the paths set down for them by the researcher. It is often alleged that the evidence of the social scientist, unlike that of the clinician or historian, which is simply 'given', is in a sense created rather than discovered. But the evidence of respondents confounds this charge.

A further reason for looking afresh at the active role of the human participants in research arises from the aspiration on the part of many social scientists and those who fund them, to make research 'useful', or helpful in the making or refinement of government, health authority or other policies. If research is to be policy relevant, then the conventional separation of observer and subjects is even more inappropriate. For until an objective criterion of needs is established, what other source of policy objectives can there be than the aspirations of policy users?

The objection to the exclusion of human participants from the business of research is therefore both epistemological and has a market and a democratic dimension. For if the human object of research and policy is a customer, then the customer is always right. And if she is a citizen, then the people are sovereign. There is a further reason why the thinking subjects of research ought wherever possible to be employed. A social or governmental policy is not applied to inert matter, but to active human beings. Its success will depend in considerable measure on its relation to their aspirations and aversions. Drawing on the active contribution of citizens to research is a necessary way of ensuring that policies which arise from that research can in a meaningful and effective way be connected with the lives of those towards whom they are directed.

Acknowledgements

My first acknowledgement must be to the women who responded to the 'Women's experiences during pregnancy' study whose comments are reproduced above. I am grateful to my colleagues Colin Pritchard and Philip Teo for permission to use the data they collected for their study, which is based at the Public Health Research Unit in Glasgow, and to Rodney Barker for his comments and advice.

Note

The Public Health Research Unit is supported by the Chief Scientist Office, Scottish Home and Health Department and the Greater Glasgow Health Board. The opinions expressed in this paper are not necessarily those of the Scottish Home and Health Department.

References

Arber, S. (1990) 'Revealing women's health: Re-analysing the General Household Survey', in H. Roberts (ed.) *Women's Health Counts*, London: Routledge.

Bagenal, F. S., Easton, D. F., Harris, E., Chilvers, C. E. D., McElwain, T. J. (1990) 'Survival of patients with breast cancer attending Bristol Cancer Help Centre', *The Lancet* 336(8715): 606–10.

Bodmer, W. (1990) 'Bristol Cancer Help Centre' (letter), *The Lancet* 336(8724): 1188.

British Journal of Obstetrics and Gynaecology (1990) 87(12).

Brown, G. H. and Harris, T. (1978) *The Social Origins of Depression: A Study of Psychiatric Disorder in Women*, London: Tavistock.

Canadian Collaborative CVS-Amniocentesis Clinical Trial Group (1989) 'Multi-centre randomised clinical trial of chorion villus sampling and amniocentesis', *The Lancet* 1(8628): 1–6.

Finch, J. (1984) ' "It's great to have someone to talk to": The ethics and politics of interviewing women', in C. Bell and H. Roberts (eds) *Social Researching: Politics, Problems and Practice*, London: Routledge & Kegan Paul.

Goodare, H. (1990) 'Bristol survey support group' (letter), *Independent on Sunday* 30 December: 16.

Graham, H. (1983) 'Do her answers fit his questions? Women and the survey method', in E. Gamarnikov, D. Morgan, J. Purvis, D. Taylorson (eds) *The Public and the Private*, London: Heinemann.

Graham, H. (1984) 'Surveying through stories', in C. Bell and H. Roberts (eds) *Social Researching: Politics, Problems, Practice*, London: Routledge & Kegan Paul.

Hayes, R. J., Smith, P. G., Carpenter, L. (1990) 'Bristol Cancer Help Centre' (letter), *The Lancet* 336(8724): 1185.

Heyse-Moore, L. (1990) 'Bristol Cancer Help Centre' (letter), *The Lancet* 336(8717): 734.

Loftus, E. F. and Fries, J. F. (1979) 'Informed consent may be hazardous to health', *Science* 204: 11.

Mason, V. (1989) *Women's Experience of Maternity Care: A Survey Manual*, London: HMSO.

Munro, J. and Payne, M. (1990) 'Bristol Cancer Help Centre' (letter), *The Lancet* 336(8717): 734.

Oakley, A. (1979) *Becoming a Mother*, Oxford: Martin Robertson.

Oakley, A. (1981) 'Interviewing women: A contradiction in terms', in H. Roberts (ed.) *Doing Feminist Research*, London: Routledge & Kegan Paul.

Oakley, A. (1990) 'Who's afraid of the randomised controlled trial? Some dilemmas of the scientific method and "good" research practice', in H. Roberts (ed.) *Women's Health Counts*, London: Routledge.

Oakley, A., McPherson, A., Roberts, H. (1990) *Miscarriage*, Harmondsworth: Penguin.

Pritchard, C. and Teo, P. (forthcoming) 'Women's experiences during pregnancy', Glasgow: Public Health Research Unit.

Roberts, H. (1981) 'Power and powerlessness in the research process', in H. Roberts (ed.) *Doing Feminist Research*, London: Routledge & Kegan Paul.

Roberts, H. (1984) 'Putting the show on the road: The dissemination of research findings', in C. Bell and H. Roberts (eds) *Social Researching: Politics, Problems, Practice*, London: Routledge & Kegan Paul.

Thomas, E. (1988) 'How doctors' secret trials abused me', *The Observer*, 9 October: 12.

Voto, L. S., Hetmanski, D. J., Broughton-Pipkin, F. (1990) 'Determinants of fetal and maternal atrial natiuretic peptide concentrations at delivery in man', *British Journal of Obstetrics and Gynaecology* 97(12): 1123–9.

Name index

Subject index